The Circadian
Prescription

The Circadian Prescription

Sidney M. Baker, M.D.
with Karen Baar, M.P.H.

A PERIGEE BOOK

A Perigee Book
Published by The Berkley Publishing Group
A division of Penguin Putnam Inc.
375 Hudson Street
New York, New York 10014

Copyright © 2000 by Sidney M. Baker, M.D.,
with Karen Baar, M.P.H.
Cover design by Walter Harper
Book design by Mauna Eichner and Lee Fukui

G. P. Putnam's Sons edition: April 2000
First Perigee edition: February 2001

Perigee ISBN: 0-399-52665-X

The Penguin Putnam Inc. World Wide Web site address is
http://www.penguinputnam.com

The Library of Congress has catalogued
the G. P. Putnam's Sons edition as follows:

Baker, Sidney M.
The circadian prescription / Sidney M. Baker, with Karen Baar.
p.   cm.
ISBN 0-399-14596-6
Includes bibliographical references and index.
1. Diet therapy.   2. Circadian rhythms.   I. Baar, Karen.   II. Title.
RM217.B3275   2000   99-053964
613.2—dc21

Printed in the United States of America

10 9 8 7 6 5 4 3 2 1

24:00
25:00
01:00
02:00
03:00
04:00
05:00
06:00
07:00
08:00
09:00
10:00
11:00
12:00
13:00
14:00
15:00
16:00
17:00
18:00
19:00
20:00
21:00
22:00
23:00
24:00
25:00
01:00

Acknowledgments

We'd both like to thank Angela Miller, without whom this happy collaboration could never have happened; John Duff, whose thoughtful, diligent editing so carefully shaped this book; Lee Fleming and Stanley Thompson for their patience, skill, and humor as they helped with data analysis and graphics development; and Lynn Sette for her research assistance. Gratitude also to the many patients who shared their stories.

KAREN BAAR AND SIDNEY M. BAKER

I dedicate this book to Cornelia Baker Mendenhall, known to me as Aunt Nel, who, from my infancy, has been a mainstay of my education and a wellspring of encouragement and example. In addition to individuals acknowledged in the text of this book I would like to give my special thanks to Jeff Bland, Ph.D., for his constant and thoughtful distillation of the current scientific literature. Years before contemplating the writing of this book I had encountered Charles Ehret, Ph.D., as an articulate lecturer with an infectious enthusiasm for puzzling out how things work. When I approached him for his help and criticism I did not anticipate the enormous generosity of his spirit and the felicity his friendship would bring to my efforts to explore and explain the research in which he has been a pioneer. The book you hold in your hand would still be a basket full of notes and dictated tapes if it were not for the partnership of my coauthor, Karen Baar. I give her my thanks for making our collaboration a crisp and productive effort that has been always harmonious and sometimes just plain fun.

SIDNEY M. BAKER

Love and gratitude to my husband, Mark Bittman, who is always my mainstay; for this project he was also my guinea pig and occasional editor. Hugs and kisses to my daughters, Emma and Kate Baar-Bittman, whose enthusiasm about my writing a book with "Dr. Sid" was contagious. Thanks also to my friends and colleagues whose interest in the book sustained me through writing, rewriting, and moments of doubt: Pamela Hort and David Paskin and their daughters Gaby and Willa, Sally Connolly, Semeon Tsalbins, Donald Margulies, Lynn Street, Kathy and Allen Mathes, John Lawrence, Jean Larson, and Katherine Grady. Extra thanks to Angela Miller and John Duff. And finally, to Sid—how lucky I am that you are not only my doctor but now also my friend—our collaboration more than met my expectations.

KAREN BAAR

24:00
25:00
01:00
02:00
03:00
04:00
05:00
06:00
07:00
08:00
09:00
10:00
11:00
12:00
13:00
14:00
15:00
16:00
17:00
18:00
19:00
20:00
21:00
22:00
23:00
24:00
25:00
01:00

Contents

SIDNEY MacDONALD BAKER, MD
WESTON, CT 06883

FOR:

Hurried Reader

℞

The Rhythmic Shake (see page 71)
Take one every morning for breakfast
for 3 weeks.

POSSIBLE SIDE EFFECTS:

Urge to read the whole book to find
out why you feel so much better

REFILLS:

As needed

LABEL AS SUCH

NJ LICENSE # 56240
BNDD AB0000000

CT LICENSE # 12263
MEDICARE DO2465

23:00
24:00
25:00
01:00
02:00
03:00
04:00
05:00
06:00
07:00
08:00
09:00
10:00
11:00
12:00
13:00
14:00
15:00
16:00
17:00
18:00
19:00
20:00
21:00
22:00
23:00
24:00
25:00
01:00

Introduction

We are not only what we eat
but when we eat.
FRANZ HALBERG

Offering the Circadian Prescription as something that works for everyone contradicts a fundamental lesson I've learned in thirty-five years of being a doctor: We are all different.

Individuality is the key that unlocks the door to the changes each of us must make to protect our health. I have spent my life taking care of *individuals,* using the tools of modern chemistry and immunology to find and treat the quirks that have gotten each one into trouble in some unique way. Yet here I am, proposing that one program is right for all of us.

Before I explain how I came to my conclusions, let me briefly point out the three main components of the Circadian Prescription. Although the program is grounded in solid scientific research, it is simple to understand and practice. Its principles are based on a fascinating web of facts and ideas that illuminate the relationship between the rhythms of your body and your harmony with the environment, a connection that is as old as life itself.

First, at the core of my program is the Circadian Diet, a simple but powerful eating plan that enables you to give your body the food it needs *when it needs it,* as dictated by the laws of circadian rhythm. Put simply, you will be eating most of your protein at breakfast and lunch and the bulk of your carbohydrates in the evening.

Second, the Circadian Diet incorporates specific foods to reduce your risk of cancer and other chronic diseases. You will be taking advantage of cutting-edge research about food, which has revealed that food is far more than a simple source of energy or a collection of nutrients; it is *information* that regulates critical biochemical processes.

With the diet as the foundation, the third component of the Circadian Prescription adds concrete techniques you can use to attain rhythmic integration, bringing into balance those body rhythms that you can control. The more integrated your rhythms, the better you will feel.

What Is Circadian Rhythm?

Research by Dr. Charles Ehret and others has revealed that human beings, like other living creatures, undergo rhythmic changes in their behavior and chemistry. These biological rhythms can be measured in body temperature, blood pressure, mental alertness, hormone and neurotransmitter production, physical strength, aerobic capacity, and countless other body functions. The rhythms are called circadian, a word derived from the Latin for "about" or "approximately" (*circa*) and "day" (*dian*). Your body's internal clock completes its rhythmic cycle *about* every twenty-four hours in synchrony with the external clock of the earth's rotation—the day and night cycle.

Not only do humans have circadian rhythms, but also these rhythms are arranged sequentially. On a farm, the farmer wakes up, milks the cows, has breakfast, feeds the chickens, and goes about his other daily chores in a certain order; if he didn't, the animals would suffer and the farm wouldn't operate smoothly. Similarly, your body performs specific biochemical activities in a regular order that's repeated every day. You couldn't function if it didn't.

Numerous experiments have shown that when left to run freely, human circadian rhythms run longer than twenty-four hours; they can and must be regularly reset to stay in harmony with the earth's cycle. Timegivers, or cues, such as light, food, and social stimulation reset your body clock every day. This flexibility of your body rhythms allows you to recover after traveling across time zones or, perhaps, working on a night shift or even staying up late, activities that disrupt your normal circadian rhythms. But the body's natural tendency is toward synchrony with the day and night cycle, and in the long run, you can't beat the clock. Staying in tune with your natural rhythms is a key to good health.

What is remarkable about circadian rhythm and the biochemical activities of the human body is that they follow the same pattern for all of us. Whether you consider yourself a "morning person" or a "night owl," your body proceeds on the same schedule as mine; we all march to the same biological drumbeat.

I'm sure you're aware of the litany of conditions that plague us all. Obesity is increasing at a dangerous rate; more than half the population in the United States is now overweight. By some estimates, insulin resistance (sometimes called hyperinsulinism or Syndrome X) affects more than one-quarter of the population in our country; this condition raises the risk for cardiovascular disease, diabetes, and chronic inflammatory problems such as colitis, arthritis, and asthma. Breast cancer threatens one in eight American women, and cancer of the prostate is a growing concern for men. And heart disease, strokes, and other so-called lifestyle diseases take a large toll.

Complaints such as fatigue, difficulty concentrating, depression, digestive and sleep disturbances, and other forms of mild malaise are less life-threatening but very common and troublesome for millions of people. The Circadian Prescription will help you tackle all of these problems. And if you are well, it is a surefire way of preserving your health and lowering your risk of serious illnesses in the future.

THE BEGINNINGS OF THE DIET

In 1971 I left my job as assistant professor of medical computer sciences at Yale Medical School to become a family doctor and pediatrician at Community Health Center Plan in New Haven, Connecticut, one of the earliest health maintenance organizations. Before that, I had practiced medicine as a medical school faculty member, a Peace Corps volunteer in Africa, and, during my training at Yale, as an intern, resident, and chief resident.

Except for a brief residency in obstetrics, my focus had always been *sick* people. But when I started working at the health plan many of my patients were essentially healthy; they simply wanted a "checkup." They had nothing amiss when I went through the standard review of systems, in which a doctor inquires about a patient's nervous, respiratory, urinary, reproductive, musculoskeletal, and digestive systems, and skin. But in my desire to get beyond the mechanical functions of my patients, I began asking them about what psychiatrists call vegetative functions, such as patterns of sleep, appetite, and elimination. Vegetative functions have to do with rhythms: sleeping at night, awakening rested and hungry, eating and eliminating on a regular schedule.

Whether or not my patients claimed to be well, I soon found that answers to questions about vegetative functions—of interest to psychiatrists as indicators of depression—revealed a lot about their health and were in and of themselves worthy targets of therapy. Even as I grew intrigued by my patients' individuality, I also realized that vegetative functions reflected ways in which people are all supposed to be the same.

A few years passed before I met Dr. Charles F. Ehret, one of the pioneers of circadian rhythm research. I had the pleasure of picking him up at the airport when he flew into New England to spend the weekend with me and a small group of holistic doctors. Our group met four times a year for weekend-long conferences in which we invited an expert to guide us through the landscape of his or her discipline with an intensity that can never be achieved in the short presentations given at medical scientific meetings.

Dr. Ehret was at the top of his field—the study of the body rhythms exhibited by creatures of various complexity—when he wrote his book *Overcoming Jet Lag,* which has since become a valuable resource for travelers crossing time zones. After our meeting, I began to adapt Dr. Ehret's guidelines for travelers on fasting, feasting, exposure to light, and use of caffeine to treatments for my patients when irregularities in their sleep, eating, and elimination patterns revealed that their circadian rhythms were out of sync.

PROTEIN IN THE MORNING AND CARBOHYDRATES AT NIGHT

Key to Dr. Ehret's advice is the *timing* of eating particular foods. Because what goes on in your body at night is completely different from what happens during the day, you require different kinds of raw materials, derived from food, for the day shift and the night shift. Protein, and the amino acids that are liberated when you digest it, supply the materials for a major biochemical cycle that occurs in the morning called adrenergic chemistry. This process is essential for creating a state of daytime alertness and activity. Without properly functioning adrenergic chemistry, you will lack energy and alertness and have difficulty concentrating, a condition we have all experienced; I call it fuzzyheaded.

On the other hand, eating carbohydrates in the evening helps your body maintain the high blood sugar level required for its nighttime activities of detoxification, repair, and restoration. When you digest carbohydrates they are broken down into sugar molecules, which travel through your bloodstream and, with the help of insulin, enter your body's cells to be burned as fuel. Not only does eating carbohydrates late in the day provide the energy your body needs for its biochemical chores to flow smoothly, but it also allows your body to absorb tryptophan and other nutrients that are needed for sleep. So eating a generous supply of carbohydrates in the evening helps you sleep better.

PRESCRIBING THE CIRCADIAN DIET: AT FIRST FOR A FEW, THEN FOR EVERYONE

Learning about circadian rhythms and the timing of foods helped me resolve a long-time quandary. Over the years, careful attention to my patients' dietary intake and a special interest in yeast allergy and fungal infections made me increasingly aware that many people with these ailments also had carbohydrate cravings and sensitivities. My friend and teacher, Dr. Orian Truss, whose initial publications on this subject attracted the attention of many doctors as well as the disapproval of many mainstream authorities, insisted that a low carbohydrate diet was essential to getting the maximum benefit from antiyeast treatments. But I argued with Dr. Truss that a low carbohydrate diet was the same as a high fat, high protein diet and therefore not a good option for the long-term dietary regimen often required by people with yeast problems.

For a long time, I remained ambivalent about diets that obliged people to eat a consistently high intake of protein and fat to the exclusion of carbohydrate, which should be a relatively large source of energy for human beings. Finally, it dawned on me that the marriage of Dr. Ehret's scientific findings with the clinical observation that many patients have carbohydrate problems could produce a compromise that would avoid extreme diets yet offer big benefits in exchange for relatively little effort.

What emerged is the Circadian Diet. I had my patients emphasize protein at breakfast and lunch and limit most of their carbohydrates to the evening. This helped them minimize the negative effects of frequent carbohydrate consumption. At the same time, *they got more benefits from whatever carbohydrates they ate because they consumed them when they were most essential to their bodies.*

The program had such a huge impact that I began prescribing it for patients with other ailments and ultimately even for those who were essentially well. The results have been remarkable. Most people get an immediate, dramatic improvement of mood and cognitive function—they feel better and are more alert—followed by gradual relief of other symptoms. The diet offers special protection against reproductive cancers in both men and women and is particularly effective for children with attention disorders and other chronic problems. And if you are concerned about your weight, you can use it as a slow, safe way to lose pounds without feeling deprived.

It is because we all have the same circadian biochemical cycles that the diet works for everyone. That is why, despite more than three decades of focusing on the individuality of my patients, I can say without hesitation that the Circadian Diet is good for *you,* whether you are a treadmiller at the gym, a vegetarian jogger, or a 1990s nutrition backlasher enjoying a glass of Côte de Rhone with your cigar in the evening.

It may reassure you to know that I personally am more of a backlasher than a fanatic. I love to eat, but I stick to the Circadian Diet because it helps me feel and function better on a day-to-day basis. Even if I weren't a physician and therefore more aware than the average guy of the bad things that can happen to people, just reading the paper and watching the news is enough to convince me that you and I are "at risk." Some of these risks, such as exposure to environmental toxins, are not easy for us to control, but there are some simple things that we can do to minimize our risk for cancer and heart disease as well as for just plain feeling crummy or not functioning up to par. The science behind the diet assures me of its protective powers, and—perhaps most important—it is not onerous to follow. The Circadian Diet combines what I know about biochemistry and rhythms with my understanding that no one wants to make the treatment worse than the problem.

You might be wondering why this important connection between diet and circadian rhythm hasn't yet reached the public, even though the scientific research has been around for a while. Most of the studies in this field have been done by researchers who have not been inclined to translate their highly scientific findings into concrete, practical applications. Since circadian research is a relatively new branch of science, its researchers have needed to have the special rigor of pioneers. Scientists involved in a new field must be especially careful to avoid the disaffection of their peers who are always on the lookout for imprecise methodology. This is a healthy state of affairs for the experts who are mapping a new territory, but there is always the danger that they become too caught up in laying down the trails to give us regular folks guided tours. This is especially true of research into circadian rhythms; this work doesn't fit neatly into any medical specialty, and doctors, who often interpret scientific research for their patients, are not familiar with it. Besides, most doctors don't know or bother much about nutrition and diet, anyway. The result? Except for jet lag and sleep disorders, mainstream medicine has virtually ignored circadian rhythms.

THE CIRCADIAN DIET, INSULIN RESISTANCE, AND CHRONIC ILLNESS

The Circadian Diet works especially well for many people who have trouble with carbohydrates. If you've ever been told that you have insulin resistance, you are one of these people. It stems from a genetic endowment gone awry.

People with insulin resistance are genetic descendants of hunter-gatherers who had the knack of being able to store fat when gathering carbohydrate-rich foods such as grass tops, seeds, berries, nuts, fruits, and roots. Ordinarily, people don't turn carbohydrates into fat. But these people were able to escalate their serum insulin levels, enhancing their capacity to store fat and becoming more efficient at conserving the energy provided by small repeated doses of carbohydrates. They were more likely to survive those times of year when carbohydrate-rich foods were scarce, giving them an evolutionary advantage.

While this capacity to raise serum insulin levels in response to carbohydrates used to be adaptive, it is a disadvantage in modern life where carbohydrates—everything from bread to pasta to soft drinks—are excessively available. Frequently escalating serum insulin levels can lead to undesirable metabolic consequences that can affect hormone chemistry, immunity, neurotransmitter function, and the utilization of fat. Among the symptoms these disruptions cause are obesity, fatigue, mood disturbances, confusion, and inflammatory illnesses such as colitis and asthma. On the Circadian Diet, you eat carbohydrates much less frequently, reducing the harmful tendency to raise serum insulin levels and the consequent results.

FOOD AS INFORMATION

Recent scientific research about food and nutrition has focused on phytonutrients (or phytochemicals), natural compounds found in plant foods that speak directly to our body chemistry, with profound effects on human health. This work has brought a new depth to our conception of what food is. In the past, food was thought to be a source of the protein, carbohydrates, and fat needed for energy as well as a provider of other nutrients, like vitamins and minerals. But food is also *information*.

Your body is an information system; your cells are constantly talking to each other through different kinds of messenger molecules. Some of the more familiar ones are neurotransmitters and hormones. When phytonutrients enter your body they join your own network of messenger molecules.

There are thousands of phytonutrients. Many are currently under investigation for their ability to prevent cancer, and they may also protect against some forms of heart disease, arthritis, and other degenerative diseases. Among the foods most intensively studied so far are soy, flaxseed, and rye fiber, whose phytonutrients provide beneficial messages that modulate your reproductive hormone chemistry and reduce the risk of cancer. The Circadian Diet shows you how to incorporate these phytonutrient-rich foods into your own diet to protect against serious chronic illnesses.

CIRCADIAN RHYTHMS AND HEALTH

A burgeoning field of research called chronobiology is revealing that circadian rhythms have a powerful impact on human functioning, health, and well-being, as well as implications for the management of medications and treatment of disease. For example:

- In the early morning hours you can be twice as sensitive to pain as you are in the late afternoon.

- Alcohol consumed late in the evening and during the night raises your blood alcohol level to a markedly greater degree than that consumed in the afternoon and early evening.

- Nighttime exposure to artificial light, which disrupts the normal circadian rhythm that triggers the release of the hormone melatonin, may be linked to an increase in breast and other cancers.

- Sleep researchers have used the hormone melatonin to restore normal twenty-four-hour sleep patterns in blind people, some of whom revert to a nearly twenty-five-hour circadian cycle because they do not receive the powerful timegiving effects of daylight and darkness.

- Jet lag and some kinds of depression, especially seasonal affective disorder (SAD), yield to treatment with appropriately timed light exposure.

- Biologists at Cornell University recently reported that they were able to reset human biological clocks by shining intense light on the back of people's knees, raising hopes for easier ways to prevent jet lag.

- Timing the intake of medications can produce more effective results. In one study, cancer researchers showed that by precisely timing the interval between the administration of the vitamin folic acid and a chemotherapy treatment they were able to increase the positive effects of chemotherapy by nearly 100 percent and also reduce toxic side effects from two- to fivefold.

- Experts in the physiology of sleep are working to develop new, safer sleep-inducing drugs using the mechanisms of circadian rhythm.

- Some experiments show that it's highly likely that your susceptibility to getting an infection is high in the early morning hours and low in the late afternoon.

RHYTHMIC INTEGRATION AND THE
CIRCADIAN PRESCRIPTION

Circadian rhythm is flexible; every day your body uses timegivers such as light, social stimulation, and food to reset your clock to coincide with the earth's twenty-four hour cycle. But this flexibility is a double-edged sword; it can cause you harm. Lack of daily exposure to direct sunlight, the unintentional effects of artificial lights at night, and the intake of caffeine, alcohol, and other drugs interfere with your body clock, throwing off your circadian rhythms in ways of which you are the unconscious victim.

The Circadian Prescription teaches you how to take advantage of your body's flexibility. While the basis of the Circadian Prescription is the diet—with special attention on the timing of protein and carbohydrates—it also includes other steps you can take to reinforce a healthy circadian rhythm.

Strengthening your circadian rhythm helps bolster other body rhythms, such as brain waves, cardiovascular tempos, breathing, and the menstrual cycle. As you support your body's chemistry and rhythmic integration, you move toward harmony with the day and night cycle. And harmony is better than disharmony.

The evidence supporting the Circadian Prescription is sturdy. It comes from three sources that, like the legs of a three-legged stool, form a support reliable enough to stand on. One important source, not always found in medical journals, are the commonsense conclusions that spring from basic facts about human circadian rhythms. Human biochemistry is rhythmic and sequential; it simply makes sense that your body will function better if given the right raw materials—carbohydrates and protein—*when they are needed.* This notion that the timing of eating positively influences the efficiency of human biochemistry is supported by the second leg of the stool, the published literature in the field of circadian physiology and rhythms.

But as a practicing physician, perhaps the strongest leg is my experience with patients. This evidence is anecdotal in the best sense of the word; it comes from my patients' stories. I can't deny that I'm predisposed to believing what my patients tell me, but thirty-five years of clinical practice has given me an eye and an ear for stories that ring true, especially when the same account comes from so many very different people. The reports I have heard—and the results I've seen—from people who have shifted to the regimen described in this book are utterly convincing. My patients' victories are what ultimately led me to share the prescription with you.

Doctors tend to use fear as a motivator, and indeed, my own personal commitment to the Circadian Prescription is based partly on my fears of cancer and other woes that could spoil my approaching old age. Success is another incentive. Seeing how my patients conquer their symptoms—and feeling so much better myself—is what keeps me doing the few simple things needed to get the benefits of the Circadian Prescription.

But knowledge is probably the strongest motivator, because it helps you gain control of your life. My career as a doctor has given me the privilege as well as the necessity of being on the lookout for my patients. I want to give them and you options that combine safe medical practices from the present with steps we can all take toward the future. I have climbed to the crow's nest to scan the medical horizon for solid grounds you can count on as the basis for improving your health and preventing illness. And I have sprinkled this book with facts and ideas that I hope will interest, amuse, and stimulate you.

I don't know if you are male or female, large, medium, or small, happy or sad, spiritually inclined or materialistic, sick or well, young or old, like me or different from me. There is one thing I am sure of, however: you have a circadian rhythm that is practically identical to mine. That is the basis for this book. Using it, you can make a small investment that will give you a tremendous return.

When you finish this book, return to this page and read the following quote from my friend and teacher Charles Ehret. It is a concise and beautiful statement of what I hope to bring you in the pages that follow:

A creature with all of its systems in strong circadian synchrony has somehow learned to "put it all together" so that the multiple environmental amenities and the magnitude of inner appetites mesh in a satiable and circadian harmony. Such fortunate creatures are rewarded by functional proficiency and longevity.[1]

How Is Your Circadian Rhythm?

Complete this questionnaire to find out whether your circadian rhythms are benefiting or suffering from things you choose to do or things that happen to you. The answers to some questions have to do with your lifestyle choices. Others reflect your body's tendency to keep to a regular rhythm.

$$
\begin{aligned}
\text{Never} &= 0 \\
\text{Rarely} &= 1 \\
\text{Sometimes, or 1 to 3 days a week} &= 2 \\
\text{Usually, or 4 to 6 days a week} &= 3 \\
\text{Always, or daily} &= 4
\end{aligned}
$$

Part 1:

_____ 1. For breakfast, I eat foods like cereal, toast, bagels, muffins, or other "bready" foods.

_____ 2. I get up in the middle of the night to eat.

_____ 3. I drink two or more caffeinated beverages (coffee, tea, soda) per day.

_____ 4. I drink a little too much alcohol more than two times per month.

Subtotal Part 1: _____

Part 2:

_____ 5. My shift rotates more than once per month.

_____ 6. I travel across at least two time zones more than once per month.

_____ 7. My shift rotation is night > evening > day.

_____ 8. I work at a job that requires me to change shifts.

Subtotal Part 2: _____

Part 3:

_____ 9. For dinner, I eat foods like pasta, rice, potatoes, and bread.

_____ 10. For breakfast, I eat foods like eggs, meat or fish, yogurt, cheese, or tofu.

_____ 11. I'm hungry for breakfast every morning.

_____ 12. I wake up feeling refreshed.

_____ 13. I have a bowel movement every morning.

_____ 14. I fall asleep easily.

Subtotal Part 3: _____

Part 4:

_____ 15. I wake up before the alarm clock goes off.

_____ 16. I have regular bowel movements when I travel.

_____ 17. I wake up at the same time every day, with or without the alarm.

_____ 18. I sleep through the night.

_____ 19. I have a bowel movement in the afternoon or evening.

_____ 20. I go to bed between 9:00 and 11:00 p.m.

Subtotal Part 4: _____

Additional Considerations (score 1 point for each if applicable):

_____ 21. I exercise for at least 20 minutes daily in an activity where I breathe regularly.

_____ 22. I exercise for at least 20 minutes at the same time every day.

_____ 23. I exercise for at least 20 minutes every afternoon.

_____ 24. I practice yoga more than three times per week.

_____ 25. I practice diaphragmatic breathing and breath control daily.

_____ 26. I am a singer, and I sing more than three times per week.

_____ 27. I play a wind instrument more than three times per week.

Additional Considerations Total: _____

Adjustment for Women Who Menstruate:

_____ 28. My periods occur every 27 to 29 days. (Add 5 points.)

_____ 29. My periods occur at irregular intervals, or not at all some months. (Subtract 5 points.)

Adjustment: _____

Your Circadian Rhythm Score

Part 1 Score _____   Part 3 Score _____

Part 2 Score _____   Part 4 Score _____

Add Part 1 and Part 2 _____   Add Part 3 and Part 4 _____

Subtract the Total Part 1 and Part 2 score
from the Total Part 3 and Part 4 score   _____

Additional Considerations score   + _____

Adjustment for Menstrual Cycle   + or − _____

Circadian Rhythm score   _____

What your Circadian Rhythm score means:

- Maximum possible score for men is 55 and for women is 60.

- Minimum possible score for men is minus 40 and for women is minus 45.

- Most people score between 30 and 40.

- Less than 20 is poor.

- 20 to 30 is below average.

- 30 to 40 is fair.

- 40 to 50 is good.

- Above 50 is excellent.

Your Active Systems Score—What You Can Change Now:

A. Add up your scores for questions 9, 10, and 21
through 27:   _____

B. Add up the scores for questions 1, 3, and 4:   + _____

Subtract B. from A. This is your Active Systems score: _____

Your Active Systems score is a measure of circadian influences that are under your control. You can increase your Active Systems score by making changes in your diet, exercising, learning to breathe diaphragmatically, and reducing your intake of caffeine and alcohol. The idea is to increase your scores to the maximum (15 points) points for the questions in part A and reduce them to zero for those in part B. And, of course, if you improve what is under your control, the other factors that make up your total Circadian Rhythm score will improve as a reflection of your efforts.

24:00
25:00
01:00
02:00
03:00
04:00
05:00
06:00
07:00
08:00
09:00
10:00
11:00
12:00
13:00
14:00
15:00
16:00
17:00
18:00
19:00
20:00
21:00
22:00
23:00
24:00
25:00
01:00

Life Is Rhythm

t's four in the morning on March 29, 1979, at Three Mile Island nuclear power plant in Pennsylvania. Bright lights illuminate a team of people and dials, switches, indicators, and gauges on walls that look like the magnified controls of a large airliner. On one dial, a team member makes a routine setting adjustment to the left instead of the right. Another dial registers a problem. Exchanges among the operators communicate small errors and misunderstandings that result in a core meltdown that comes within a whisker of depopulating a large part of the northeastern United States.[1] In 1986 the Chernobyl meltdown did result in the depopulation and radiation poisoning of a large area of the Ukraine—the biggest nuclear disaster in history.

Both incidents, along with hundreds of close calls in the nuclear power industry and real disasters in aviation, shipping, and industry, were the result of human error. Take away the human factor, and nuclear power plants and many other machines, computers, devices, and systems would rarely fail. Factor in human error, and failure is bound to happen. Blame falls on the operators, the pilot, the driver, the programmer, or the night watchman. They are all human and, like each of us, can slip up from time to time.

It's just a matter of chance. Or is it? The real error at Three Mile Island was the fault not of the operators who got the blame but of the managers who assigned them an inhuman work schedule. Not cruelly inhuman but ignorantly inhuman, because the schedule ignored a fundamental human condition: circadian rhythm.

Ignorance of circadian rhythm has consequences that range from enormous disasters like Three Mile Island to dropping a carton of milk on the kitchen floor when you are already running late to disturbances in your health and well-being. Even if you don't work at a nuclear power plant at 4:00 a.m., disruptions of your circadian timing can cause disasters for you.

Circadian Rhythm

The term "circadian" was coined by Franz Halberg, a scientist at the University of Minnesota, whose research showed that blood count in animals varied according to a strict rhythm that coincided with a cycle that was a little longer than the twenty-four-hour day and night cycle. He abandoned the old term "diurnal," which meant exactly a day, and introduced the new term, "circadian." The word entered our vocabulary when he published a paper in 1959—quite recently, considering that the term describes a fundamental quality that has been part of all living things for billions of years.[2]

Circadian rhythms have now been the subject of comprehensive scientific study for more than three decades. In humans, blood count, temperature and most other measurements of body chemistry, hormone secretion, mood, attentiveness, visual acuity, physical strength, digestive secretion, even rate of hair growth change from hour to hour. If you measure any function at 8:00 a.m., for instance, and mark it on a piece of paper, put the 9:00 a.m. measurement next to it and continue this process every hour for a day, the points you have marked, once joined, will look like a wave, as in the following graphs. The wave will have its crest at a certain time in the twenty-four-hour span and its trough at another. The peaks and valleys occur at different times depending on what you measure, but they are almost precisely the same for all people. For example, the highest point of body temperature may be in the evening while the pinnacle of cortisone-type hormones in the blood is in the morning hours. The sharpness of the peaks also differs. After midnight the tip of the sleep hormone melatonin is a tall spike, whereas the daily rise and fall of your white blood count is a gentle wave.

The complex interaction of all your body's functions is like the har-

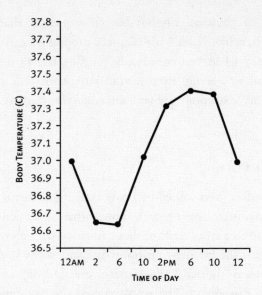

Body temperature is at its lowest at 6:00 a.m. and peaks at 6:00 p.m.

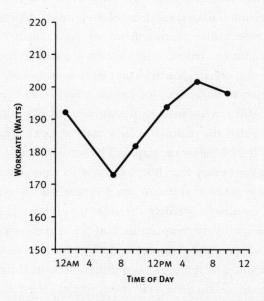

The peak of your capacity for performing muscular activities occurs just a little after 6:00 p.m.

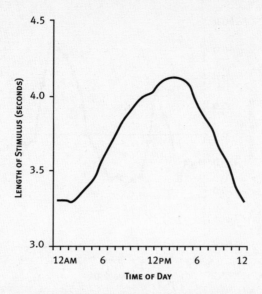

If you're going to the dentist, consider a late afternoon appointment.
You can best tolerate pain from cold and other stimuli in the mid- to late afternoon.

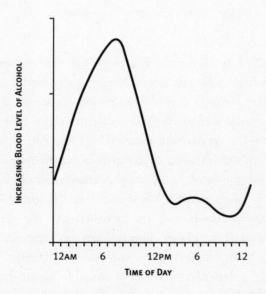

Based on the level of blood alcohol that occurs after equal doses of alcohol
taken at different times of day and night, your body is much more able to
metabolize alcohol between 2:00 and 10:00 p.m. than at other times.

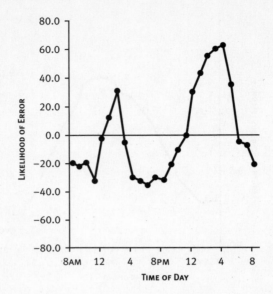

People encounter problems when expected to perform dangerous tasks at times of day or night when circadian rhythms put them at a disadvantage. In the early afternoon your chance of making mistakes is about 50 percent higher than before noon or in the early evening. Four a.m. is the time when real disasters occur and is associated with a nearly 100 percent increase in the incidence of work disasters.

monious sound of an orchestra. The players in this orchestra are your body's one hundred trillion cells, and Nature is the conductor. The most conspicuous ways Nature marks the tempo are the annual rhythm of the earth's voyage around the sun, the moon's twenty-eight-day cycle, and the earth's rotation—the twenty-four-hour cycle of day and night, within all of which your body chemistry and its innate circadian cycles operate.

Scientists use the word "circa" (approximately) in discussing human body rhythms because research has shown that the internal body clock runs longer than twenty-four-hours, in contrast to the precise twenty-four-hour rotation of our planet. This rhythm was measured in many experiments in which people lived, sometimes for months, in caves or chambers specially designed to be free of any clues about the time of day in the real world. At the beginning of these experiments the subjects' entrainment to the day and night cycle was reinforced by regular exposure to light, food, activity, and exercise. They entered isolation with a strong twenty-four-hour cycle, which shifted as their innate rhythm emerged in the absence of environmental timegivers. This rhythm is very precise in each individual. It is the same "day" after "day," understanding that in this case "day" refers to the repetitive cycle of the individual, which, according to most research, runs within a few minutes of twenty-five hours. (Recently one of the foremost circadian researchers has claimed that the human body clock runs closer to 24.2 hours. This finding is likely to be vigorously challenged by other researchers, and their discussion will certainly percolate down to the daily news. Meanwhile, this debate has no practical impact on the Circadian Prescription.)[3]

It isn't really known why the internal clock of the human body runs longer than twenty-four-hours. It may be that our clocks were established in the remote past when planetary timing was slower. In any case, given the appropriate cues—food, light, and social stimulation—the body's cycle resets itself every day to a twenty-four-hour rhythm in harmony with Nature.

CIRCADIAN RHYTHMS AND YOUR HEALTH

Your body's flexibility is, in some ways, a gift. It lets you accommodate changes like the shift in time zones you encounter when you travel. But there is a limit to your ability to adapt. Some of us are born with more tolerance for the stresses and strains that come with shifting our activities away from the normal rhythm, but there are no real night owls. People who have jobs where they work all night when they should be resting and sleep during the day when they should be active have a hard time adjusting; some research shows that they never completely get used to this reversal of the day and night cycle. Night shift workers more frequently have disturbed sleep patterns, and they also suffer from an increased incidence of cardiovascular disease, mood disorders, and gastrointestinal ailments.[4] The consequences of being out of synchrony with natural rhythms can be dire, as in the example of Three Mile Island.

But abuses of circadian rhythm are not always so obvious. The human body is so beautifully orchestrated—and adaptable—that it's easy to be unaware of timing and its critical effects on body chemistry. Still, you pay a price when you don't keep the beat. A growing body of scientific knowledge about the presence and power of body rhythms is showing that they are profoundly important no matter what your activities. For example, even the one-hour time shifts that occur when changing to or from Daylight Savings time are connected to a significant increase in traffic accidents.[5]

In the future, your doctor may consider circadian rhythms in many aspects of the care you receive, based on scientific evidence now available or in the pipeline. But you don't have to wait for that because right now you can begin to apply some elementary rules that I have found successful in my medical practice. With the Circadian Diet you can anticipate what will eventually be common knowledge by making simple changes to synchronize your diet with the needs of your circadian chemistry and harmonize the activities of your body and mind with the timing of day and night. What you eat matters, but the timing of when you eat protein and carbohydrates also has consequences for your short- and long-term health.

THE DIETARY IMPLICATIONS OF CIRCADIAN RESEARCH

During the 1960s and 1970s, talented scientists, such as Dr. Charles Ehret of Argonne National Laboratory in Illinois,[6] conducted studies to unravel the mysteries of circadian chemistry. Some of this work was sponsored by the United States military, which has a keen interest in human performance requiring a clear head and good reflexes, especially when it comes to air transport of troops. The military moves personnel across many time zones and, particularly in crisis situations, these soldiers must be able to deal with the impact of jet lag—a disruption of circadian rhythms—without the luxury of time to adapt.

Dr. Ehret's research began with the observation of the growth cycles of tiny organisms, then progressed to studying the details of the day and night cycle in various animals and, ultimately, in soldiers. It turned out that the most effective measures for manipulating the body's rhythms to counteract jet lag and shift work fatigue were exposure to light, caffeine, and food, with special attention to the timing of protein and carbohydrate intake. The researchers found that the body's daytime chemical chores benefit from a generous quantity of protein. On the other hand, nighttime chemical activities require an abundant supply of the energy and signals provided by carbohydrates. What is remarkable about these findings is that they follow the same pattern for everyone.

Yet most people feed their bodies exactly the opposite of what circadian rhythm demands. Cereal, pancakes, bread, bagels, muffins, donuts, juice—all high carbohydrate foods—are the most popular breakfast items. And in recent years, concern about cholesterol as well as busy schedules have relegated high protein traditional foods such as eggs and breakfast meats to weekends or to the "forbidden" list. Sandwiches, fries, and chips are commonplace at lunch, and although the pattern is changing, dinners still consist primarily of high protein fare like fish, chicken, and meat.

Individuality, including food preferences, makes it hard to apply the same rules to everyone—Jack Sprat could eat no fat; his wife could eat no lean. Your meat may be someone else's poison. And dietary traditions may be even harder to overcome. But the Circadian Diet uses science to provide a better way of eating *regardless of who you are,* allowing you to feel better, be healthier, stay young and beautiful longer, and reduce the risk of cancer, especially in your reproductive system. Although its approach is scientific, it can be just as easy and enjoyable as the way you've eaten in the past.

The Circadian Diet uses scientific understanding to introduce the impact of timing on what you eat. It does this in two ways. First, we now know that we are all rhythmically the same, so if there's something about eating that has to do with rhythms, it can safely be recommended for anyone. Second, scientific research has helped us see the invisible circadian rhythms that govern what is happening from moment to moment in our internal chemistry and to tailor our diets accordingly.

MEETING YOUR BODY'S NEEDS—DAY AND NIGHT

If you could look through a window into your body you would see that what goes on there during the day is totally different from what happens at night. Every day your body goes through a sequence of biochemical operations in which specific functions occur at particular times and not at others. You probably know that at certain times of the day you tend to be sleepier or that at other times you can think more clearly or exercise more successfully. This is because you are obeying a fundamental rhythm of human chemistry that is not only obvious to the ordinary person but can also be demonstrated by various clinical measures. Science provides us with a deeper understanding. It is just as important to match other activities, particularly eating, to the same schedule of chemistry so you can provide the necessary materials demanded by specific processes that are going on in your body day and night.

You don't have to be a scientist to understand that you can't go looking for owls during the day because owls are active at night; nor do you hunt for particular butterflies at night, because they are sleeping after their daytime activities of visiting day-nectaring plants. By the same token, it's pointless to look in your body during the day for certain hormones, like melatonin, that are active at night or to search in the evening for cortisol, a hormone that is active early in the morning. Naturally, you're not really concerned about whether you can find specific chemicals in your body. But you should be concerned about how you feed the chemistry that allows these substances to be made at the right time in the twenty-four-hour cycle.

I've already mentioned that the body operates in waves. These waves follow a specific order. Just as in a piece of music, there are parts that flow in a particular sequence. If you could look into your liver, brain, or other vital organs as you read these lines you would find them doing certain chores—making hormones and neurotransmitters or preparing toxins for safe disposal, for example. Once completed, these tasks will be placed on hold and others will begin. The scheduling of these myriad chemical processes is so complicated that it would be a full-time job for you and a small staff of assistants to monitor it. Even then, you'd never be able to keep track of it all. Luckily, Nature has provided you with an internal metronome that keeps everything on tempo.

The good news is that the complex scheduling of your body's rhythmic activities, like breathing, is so automatic you don't have to consciously run it. The bad news is that neglecting its importance can get you in trouble. You probably know that you should sleep at night and be awake during the day; when you break this rule there can be hell to pay. If you could sense what's going on inside your body at a cellular level as easily as you sense when you need to sleep at night, then you would know that the rhythmic rules of your body's chemistry call for an emphasis on certain foods for fuel and information at certain times.

I'll tell you more about how this works in the following chapters. For now, to optimize your circadian harmony, you need only remember that the work your body does in the morning requires raw materials that are provided by protein and that nighttime chores need carbohydrates.

You can't really hear the music of the orchestra that is your body. But science tells us that there is a sequence, a beat, a rhythm. When you're healthy, members of the orchestra play in harmony; when that harmony is missing, health deteriorates. Eating is the single most important activity in which you engage where timing is important. That's why diet is the cornerstone of the Circadian Prescription.

Some of you may be inclined to follow the Circadian Diet more strictly than others, and I certainly encourage some flexibility. No one, however, is an exception to the rule that this is the way to eat. When it comes to rhythms, we are all the same. No matter how we differ, we all live on the same planet and dance to its beat. Understanding how the timing of what you eat helps you obey this rhythm is crucial to achieving the harmony that produces good health.

If you're skeptical that the same diet can be right for everyone, you're not alone. I had my doubts, too. In the next chapter I'll explain how the Circadian Diet challenged thirty-five years of practicing medicine based on every patient's individuality.

24:00
25:00
01:00
02:00
03:00
04:00
05:00
06:00
07:00
08:00
09:00
10:00
11:00
12:00
13:00
14:00
15:00
16:00
17:00
18:00
19:00
20:00
21:00
22:00
23:00
24:00
25:00
01:00

CHAPTER

2

The Paradox of Individuality

My job is practicing medicine—which means listening to my patients' stories. My role in these conversations is to filter scientific research to make it understandable enough to meet the needs of my patients and make the proposed remedies easy to do. When I started out as a doctor, I didn't think that dietary changes could be important remedies. Yet the more I have learned about nutrition, the more I've become convinced of its curative powers and the more disconcerted I am by the scientific disputes and public confusion about food and nutrition.

My response to patients' stories, and what I'm telling you here, is that the Circadian Diet *is* a dependable and clear message about nutrition that can be gleaned from the scientific research in recent decades. Yet to someone with my training and experience, the diet poses this paradox: I am more impressed than most doctors by the need for individualizing treatment, including diet, but circadian rhythm is a universal rule that is just as powerful as individuality. While every patient is different, some share your problems, and all share with you the benefits of translating circadian science about your body's day and night cycle into simple changes that make a big difference.

Mary Jo Page is warm and wise with a rare depth that I think comes from the difficulties of raising a child with problems. A native Southerner, she also has an appearance of health and attractiveness that might remind you of a homecoming queen (she was the runner-up). I first got to know

Mary Jo about five years ago when she brought her daughter Annie to see me for delays in her speech and mental development.

Mary Jo herself became my patient when she was forty-two. She had always been healthy, but she had started feeling tired, spacey, and generally unwell. She had developed a list of nasty symptoms, including bloating, severe indigestion, hair loss, weight gain, dizzy spells, heart palpitations, and frequent colds. Her menstrual cycle, which had always been twenty-eight days long, had shortened to twenty or twenty-one days, and she had an itchy, scaly rash on her chin and forehead. Although the problems seemed unconnected, they had all started after she'd stopped—"cold turkey," as she said—her regular high consumption of diet cola. This was the only clue that linked her symptoms.

Mary Jo is the only person I know who developed negative symptoms after discontinuing diet soda. Usually it is just the other way around. I cannot say whether she might have gotten rid of her symptoms by drinking diet soda again. But I wouldn't recommend it, because artificial sweeteners exert an unwelcome trickery on blood sugar mechanisms by promising sweetness (carbohydrates) when none is delivered.

As I do with every patient, I asked Mary Jo about her diet. She was eating a bagel and a banana for breakfast, sandwiches for lunch, and *lots* of diet cola; in short, a great deal of carbohydrates. I recommended that she change her diet to include higher proportions of protein in the morning and hold off on eating carbohydrates until after 4:00 p.m.

She responded dramatically to my simple prescription. She knew within two days that we were on the right track, although it took a week until she could avoid carbohydrates until the late afternoon without feeling lightheaded. She started losing weight immediately, and her symptoms began to clear up. Today, still on the Circadian Diet (although she cheats once in a while), her symptoms are gone. And she says: "I feel better than ever. I'm not hungry in the late morning any more, and for the first time in my life I don't crave sugar."

Mary Jo's success in relieving a wide range of symptoms—gastrointestinal disturbances, weight gain, food cravings, skin rashes, disruption in her menstrual cycle, fatigue, spaciness, and a general feeling of malaise—has been repeated with countless other patients who have achieved similar results from making the *same* dietary changes. While my respect for the uniqueness of each patient has only increased over thirty-five years of practicing medicine, I have come to understand that there is something I can prescribe for *all* my patients: the Circadian Diet.

WE ALL ARE DIFFERENT

When I was a medical student my professors encouraged me to become a teacher and researcher, saying that everyday practice would be boring. Yet after many years of taking care of patients I am sure that nothing could be less routine than the constant challenge of determining what it might take to help a patient get better or stay well. The challenge is that each person is unique; even identical twins who share the same genetic code are different in many ways.

No two people have the identical response to a particular stress or a given treatment. In my effort to be a good doctor I am bound to respect the individuality of a patient's symptoms even when they are similar to those of other patients. I often think that good medical treatment is like custom tailoring. We measure and try it on, measure and try it on again and keep it up until we get the right fit.

Naming a problem, or in other words, having a diagnosis, can be a big help in directing treatment, especially in acute illnesses, whether it's chickenpox, strep throat, food poisoning, or poison ivy, where a sudden or short-term problem responds to the same treatment in most people. With chronic illness, however, the story is different. Simply pronouncing the name of the illness—depression, colitis, asthma, dermatitis—isn't a sufficient basis for a remedy. This is especially troublesome when it comes to those diagnoses where little is known about how to treat the condition. For years, I have been especially interested in the plight of people who have been told by their doctors: "I know what you've got, and there's not much you can do about it."

But as long as you understood the notion that your illness, whatever its label, might have any of a number of causes that are specific to you, you'd recognize that there is a lot that can be done. For example, a sensitivity to wheat can trigger colitis, arthritis, or depression, depending on the individual. The opposite is also true: one disease can have any number of causes. A child with attention deficit disorder may have a food allergy or a metabolic abnormality, or he may simply be assigned to a grade appropriate for his age and IQ but too high for his developmental age. Nowhere has my individualized approach been more rewarding than when it's successful in treating the difficulties encountered by children who fail to thrive in their development and learning.

Over the past three decades I have focused on the immunologic and biochemical details that frequently explain the mysteries of chronic illness and sometimes require very different treatments for people with similar symptoms. "Immunologic" and "biochemical" may sound fancy, but what I mean is simple. If you came to see me, the map I'd use to treat you would come down to two simple questions that I ask myself and teach my patients to ask when confronting a puzzling illness. First, is there something from the environment—a germ, a toxin, or an allergen—that doesn't agree with you in some particular way and that, if eliminated, would relieve your symptoms? Second, is there something for which you have a special need because of a unique quirk in your biochemistry? It could be a vitamin, mineral, amino acid, fatty acid or other nutritional supplement, light, or perhaps the most important nutrient, love. Using this map as my guide, I apply the tools of laboratory medicine, common sense, and dialogue to find out as much as I can. I've found that I often get results with illnesses that didn't yield well to my former more mainstream approach, in which I was taught to name the disease and then prescribe the same drug for anyone with its symptoms.

I started out this chapter by telling you that the Circadian Diet works for everyone. But it doesn't help everyone in the same way. What happened with Annie differs from her mother Mary Jo's story. Remember, I was trying to help Annie with delayed speech and mental development. As part of my strategy of tailoring a treatment to fit her unique immunological and biochemical size and shape, I had already investigated her allergies and special needs for nutrients. Now, I suggested that she try a change in her diet. She was to have a heavy load of protein at breakfast and lunch with most of her carbohydrate intake in the evening. I was trying to remedy two problems with this approach. First, Annie had carbohydrate cravings. Second, even though her spaciness had different causes from that of her mother and other children whose attention and alertness had been improved by the Circadian Diet, I thought the diet had a good chance of helping to sharpen her focus.

Unfortunately, the diet didn't help Annie much with her mental development. Like me, you might find this discouraging. Clearly, if you try the Circadian Diet and benefit as Mary Jo did, I won't have to convince you of its merits. But even if, like Annie, you fail to realize rapid and noticeable changes from the diet or if you're already feeling so good there's no room for improvement, I am still convinced that the circadian approach to eating is good for you. Although effective medical treatment usually gives you some fairly immediate response so that your body says, "Thanks, that makes me feel much better," there are important exceptions; for these treatments, the payoff is long term. Besides bringing dramatic alleviation of symptoms in more than one-half of the people who try it, the Circadian Diet leads to better health and vitality for everyone in the long run because it lowers the risk for certain cancers and other serious illnesses.

My confidence in the diet is based on this paradox: While we are all different biochemically and deserve custom tailoring of our medical treatment, we are all the same rhythmically. We are all bound by the same need to time the kinds of food we eat just as we all should obey the more obvious need to be awake during the day and sleep at night.

DIETARY TIMING AND CIRCADIAN RHYTHMS

Whenever a doctor starts to talk about eating, people expect to be told what to eat or avoid. But the Circadian Diet doesn't change *what* you eat—assuming you're eating a healthy variety of foods—as much as it changes *when* you eat it. What I suggested to Annie and her mom was not complicated. They should eat a high protein breakfast and lunch, saving any large amounts of carbohydrates for the evening.

How you time the intake of certain foods is important because your body's daily biochemical routines are divided into multiple segments. Scientists have learned that many chemical processes in the body occur in a very narrow time slot. It's as if a certain department, say in your liver, works on a particular chore from 4:00 p.m. to 5:00 p.m. Then the biochemical workers on that chore are told: "Shop's closed. Go home. Come back tomorrow at 4:00 p.m. Now the guys on the next shift are coming in to do their job."

What's more, many of these biochemical processes have their own circadian rhythms, and each of these activities has a time of day when it happens with particular intensity. I think of living in sync with these processes as "riding the wave of time" because the body's chemistry operates in waves. It can be surveyed by various measures—like temperature or blood chemistry—of the ripples, waves, breakers, and swells that take place over time intervals of seconds, minutes, hours, days, months, seasons, years, and cycles of years. Your health depends on whether you ride your body's waves or get knocked over by them. Just as a good surfer catches a wave at the right moment, when you synchronize your activities to match the natural cycles of time you get a better ride in life.

CATCHING THE WAVE

Catching the wave has implications for the timing of both positive and negative influences on your health. Research on animals (which are the same as humans in this regard) has shown that if a substance that interferes with the chemistry of adrenaline is given during the daytime rise in body temperature, the substance acts as a poisonous disrupter of the body's rhythms. Such disrupters are called dyschronogens by research scientists. The same substance given during the hours when body temperature is falling (during the night for humans) causes no disruption because the targeted adrenaline chemistry is inactive at that time. Since the substance involved is L-dopa, a medication used to treat the human condition of Parkinsonism, knowing how to catch these waves has an especially poignant human relevance.[1]

The body's circadian rhythm has nothing to do with so-called biorhythms, which are cycles over periods of weeks that are supposed to begin at birth and continue throughout life in ways that make certain days more or less disposed to success or problems with various tasks. Despite interesting examples of individuals for whom achievement or catastrophe coincided with the day predicted by their biorhythm chart, there is no scientific evidence to support the notion of biorhythms.

In the future your health and that of your children and grandchildren will be improved by advances in scientific understanding of how the many circadian rhythms of the body can be made more harmonious. Learning to synchronize the intake of various medications, nutrients, and other stimuli with the timing of chemical and electrical events in the body will be a major aspect of healing; in fact this work is already underway in the fields of chronobiology and chronopharmacology.

Of all the rhythms that affect your life, the day and night cycle is the most significant. And the most important of all activities in this regard, and one over which you have the most control, is eating. So for now, you can relax about all of those other waves and take confidence in the already established importance of the dietary timing of proteins and carbohydrates. Starting today, you can synchronize your bodily rhythms with the natural flow of time.

UNDERPINNINGS OF THE DIET

What really inspires my enthusiasm for the Circadian Diet is the following set of facts. First, diets that require people to make *major* changes in the way they eat are too hard to maintain. Second, extreme diets usually don't make much sense because human beings are not meant to survive on dietary extremes in the long run.

Third, there is abundant scientific evidence that much of the chronic illness in our culture stems from eating too many carbohydrates.[2] The negative effects of carbohydrate overload are reflected in high serum insulin levels and damage to fat metabolism that most people these days lump under the heading of "cholesterol." In fact, cholesterol is not so great a culprit when its effects are compared to the bad effects of carbohydrates.

When it comes to carbohydrates, it's really more a question of frequency than of quantity, unless you are pigging out on candy and other sweets, junk foods, soft drinks, and alcohol or your primary goal is weight loss. The key to improving your health is to consume carbohydrates less frequently, one of the cornerstones of the Circadian Diet. Less frequently means once a day. When should that once a day be? In the evening. The evidence for the benefits of evening consumption of carbohydrates is well established, particularly in scientific studies showing the need for carbohydrates to support the nighttime chemistry of the body.[3]

Just as important as consuming carbohydrates in the evening is eating protein in the morning and at lunch. Scientific research shows that morning protein supplies the raw materials necessary for the body's daytime biochemical activities. There is also good scientific evidence showing that the body efficiently sets aside protein taken during the day that is required for nighttime chores.[4, 5] (I discuss protein further in chapter 5.)

When you eat carbohydrates and protein is critical to following the Circadian Diet, but it's also important to pay attention to *what* you eat. Certain foods are particularly rich in constituents called phytochemicals that promote health in a variety of ways.

These are the underpinnings; read on to find out more about how they work.

23:00
24:00
25:00
01:00
02:00
03:00
04:00
05:00
06:00
07:00
08:00
09:00
10:00
11:00
12:00
13:00
14:00
15:00
16:00
17:00
18:00
19:00
20:00
21:00
22:00
23:00
24:00
25:00
01:00

CHAPTER

3

Food Is Information:
Phytonutrients and Natural Rhythms

Until two hundred years ago most of the rules of eating had to do with avoiding things that we assumed were bad for us, yet we weren't very well informed about the goodness in food beyond questions of taste, texture, and freshness. In all human endeavors, the 1800s could have been called the energy century. As the burning of coal and later petroleum fueled the Industrial Revolution, scientists also explored the basis for food's capacity to yield energy and came to understand its three basic components: protein, fat, and carbohydrates.

Further study revealed that food contains other substances besides protein, fat, and carbohydrates that add value to what we eat—the vitamins, minerals, fatty acids, and amino acids that aid in the burning of our metabolic fire while protecting us from its sparks. And today researchers continue to study the differences in individual needs for these nutrients as well as their potential to prevent illness.

Appropriately for our era, the information age, we now know that in addition to calories, vitamins, minerals, and other nutrients, food contains information. Human chemistry is an information system; the cells that make up your body talk to each other constantly through the chemical transfer of messages in hormones, neuropeptides, neurotransmitters, and prostaglandins. Not all these messengers are created in your body; some, called phytonutrients, come from the plant foods in your diet. The phytonutrients in soy, flaxseed, and certain other foods are substances that provide especially helpful information to enhance well-being and reduce your risk of disease.

PHYTOCHEMICALS

The word *phytochemicals* combines *phyto,* meaning plant, and *chemical,* meaning a basic or simple substance. Phytochemicals or phytonutrients, as they are sometimes called, are plant-derived substances that interact with your chemistry to enhance or harm your body's capacity to send and receive internal chemical messages such as hormones and neurotransmitters. In recent times, thanks to a big leap in the science of nutrition, we've learned that there is more to eating than consuming calories and nutrients. The term "phytochemicals" recognizes that food can potentially influence body chemistry in major ways previously thought possible only with drugs.

23:00
24:00
25:00
01:00
02:00
03:00
04:00
05:00
06:00
07:00
08:00
09:00
10:00
11:00
12:00
13:00
14:00
15:00
16:00

What does all this have to do with rhythm? These plant-derived nutrients permit animals to stay in synchrony with the seasons. You are healthiest when you live in harmony with the cadence of many rhythms. Circadian rhythm is the most obvious, but other examples include the monthly menstrual cycle as well as the yearly rotation of spring, summer, winter, and fall.

LIGHT, PLANTS, AND THE SEASONAL RHYTHMS

Imagine a time in the distant past when all living things consisted of only one cell. At the beginning, this cell was presumably naked, that is, colorless with a transparent membrane that exposed its internal workings to the rays of the sun. In order for naked cells to make effective use of sunlight and defend themselves against the potentially injurious effects of sunburn, they created colored substances that absorbed light in a protective or a constructive fashion. Such colored substances, or pigments, are familiar to you in at least one example—chlorophyll, the green pigment found in the leaves of plants that absorbs sunlight and arranges for its transformation into sugars. As time passed, the growing variety and intricacy of cells and the eventual development of multicellular creatures was associated with an increasing complexity of pigments that were then and still are needed to protect cells from their environment.

The part of a plant that most requires protection is the seed, which falls to the ground and lies in soil until it germinates. The soil is full of bacteria that defend themselves by secreting toxins into the soil to scare off any competitors. They also survive by reproducing at a rapid clip. The seed is obviously part of a much slower reproductive cycle, which may take a whole year, as opposed to twenty minutes for a bacterium. The protection that a seed needs from the surrounding bacteria is afforded by a variety of substances that are embedded in its outer structure, including parts of the fiber that holds the seed together.

Some of the benefit that you get from eating the whole grain, the whole flaxseed, and the whole soybean is defense against harmful bacteria or fungal rot. You also get the protection against the sun that the seed made for itself in the form of antioxidants.

But the most important thing you get from the seeds is information about the environment in which they were grown. While much of this has yet to be fully understood by scientists, the part of the information system that has been explored most fully deals with communication about one critical aspect of the environment—time.

Light is one of the most important timekeepers for animals and humans. This is particularly true in the northern latitudes, where there are marked seasonal shifts in the length of day and, therefore, the exposure of living things to light and dark and heat and cold, all of which have a major impact on the plans any animal might have for reproduction.

Plant pigments embody messages about these changing effects of light. When animals eat plants, these messages go to their reproductive systems, giving them information about the change of seasons. This helps them synchronize their life cycles to the cycles of nature so they conceive and give birth at the most auspicious time.

Take a minute and watch my wife Natalia's two pet goats in the meadow. They are browsers, not grazers, so they do not mow the lawn; in fact, they have a strong taste for expensive shrubs such as roses and magnolia. In the meadow, even if supplied on a daily basis with all of their favorite foods, they persist in sampling a great variety of plants. A little poison ivy here (not at all poisonous to goats), some grass there, topped off by tastes of barberry, maple, goldenrod, chokecherry, grape, Virginia creeper, white lettuce, bull briar, Japanese honeysuckle, wild sorrel, bittersweet, moss, hickory, and raspberry. Besides a number of plant compounds that presumably are good for goats, the wild food brings them messages about the season. Every day, every week, every month, the plants have a different taste and chemical composition. They are providing signals of the changing seasons that the goats can use to plan their reproductive lives.

We humans share much of our body chemistry with animals. But we act as if we don't have to play by the same rules when it comes to maintaining our physical health. For example, you live in a heated house, use artificial light that permits you to stay up at night, and are relatively indifferent to the time of year when planning your pregnancies. If you consumed a "normal" diet, I would leave you alone and wish you well in your food-gathering. The normal diet that I'm talking about is the diet of your ancestors who lived more than ten thousand years ago. They got up every morning and went looking for food in a natural environment where there were no farms. They ate what was available in the fields, forests, oceans, beaches, and rivers where they lived.

If you ate a similar diet, it would include a rich variety of animal and plant foods. The plant foods in particular would bring you a constant supply of messages about what is happening in the natural world around you. Unfortunately, most Americans do not eat a particularly varied diet. United States Department of Agriculture dietary surveys show that only 52 percent of Americans reach the maximum score for variety; this maximum is based on eating only eight different foods in one given day. If you ate the same eight foods every day, you would still reach the highest score. Moreover, the score ranks all foods equally. For example, french fries count as potatoes, and the apples in apple pie count as fruit. Americans tend to include a great many processed foods in their diets and to exclude fresh, whole plant foods, depriving themselves of the beneficial messages these foods contain.[1]

If modern-day human behavior is not so closely tied to food intake, why do these messages matter? You share with all animals a legacy that enables various plant substances to continue to have profound positive effects on the hormonal chemistry of your reproductive system. Not getting these messages has a negative effect on your reproductive health, regardless of your body's relationship to seasonal planning. Disease is the price you pay.

ISOFLAVONES AND LIGNANS

Modern science has identified particular phytonutrients, called isoflavones and lignans, which can bring you the reproductive health benefits enjoyed by your ancestors. Dr. Herman Adlercreutz, a leader among researchers studying these phytonutrients, has documented that people who consume moderate amounts of soy protein, rye fiber, or flaxseed, all of which contain isoflavones and lignans, have reduced rates of reproductive cancers and other diseases. Besides reducing the risk of reproductive cancer, these phytonutrient-rich foods also contribute to an overall improvement in reproductive function.[2]

Dr. Adlercreutz's work has also revealed the precise way in which the protein in soy as well as substances derived from the fiber in flaxseed, rye, and other seeds play a role in human biochemistry. Parts of the soy protein are released during digestion and transformed by germs that live in your digestive tract into molecules that bring messages to your body. These messages affect cell division and the growth of blood vessels. They also help regulate sex hormones, such as estrogen and testosterone.

Unlike other animals, humans no longer need to learn from phytonutrients what season is coming next. But the influence of plant foods on the

23:00
24:00
25:00
01:00
02:00
03:00
04:00
05:00
06:00
07:00
08:00
09:00
10:00
11:00
12:00
13:00
14:00
15:00
16:00
17:00
18:00
19:00
20:00
21:00
22:00
23:00
24:00

GERMS

When I refer to germs I mean bacteria and fungi, but in general the term may include any of the following infectious agents: prions, viruses, bacteria, fungi, or protozoa. Germs may be good guys or bad guys, depending on the situation. As you will see, getting benefits from your diet depends not only what you eat but on how the food is handled by beneficial germs that live in your digestive tract. However tiny germs may be, their capacity for complex chemistry outdistances our own. Paradoxically, the bigger and more complicated the organism—and human beings are at the top of the list—the smaller is its capacity for certain vital biochemical processes.

People think of germs as things to be avoided, and indeed, most human illnesses result from germs. But as you read this book I hope you will sharpen your ear for news that you will be hearing more and more in the next few years about the need to feed and protect the *friendly* germs that can make the difference between success and failure for a good diet.

reproductive rhythms of animals provides the context for understanding how, and perhaps why, plant foods like soybeans, rye fiber, and flaxseed continue to affect our reproductive health.

EASING REPRODUCTIVE PROBLEMS
WITH PHYTONUTRIENTS

For my patients who include soy, flaxseed, and rye in their diets, I've seen dramatic positive changes in those whose reproductive troubles fall far short of cancer. In fact, I believe these foods are helpful for people who have just about anything wrong with their endocrine systems. By endocrine I'm referring to the whole array of body functions that are governed by substances called hormones, particularly the reproductive or steroid hormones such as estrogen, progesterone, dehydroepiandrosterone (DHEA), testosterone, and pregnenolone.

I hear frequently from my women patients that a gynecologist has responded to their symptoms—ranging from breast tenderness, lumpy breasts, irregular menstrual cycles, premenstrual tension, menstrual cramps, and fluid retention during various phases of the menstrual cycle to infertility and menopausal symptoms such as hot flashes—with a shrug and the statement: "It's something wrong with your hormones." This diagnosis, or more accurately, lack of diagnosis, comes after the doctor has determined that there is no serious contributing factor—a tumor, preg-

---

PHYTOESTROGENS

The term "phytoestrogen," which often appears interchangeably with the words "phytochemical" and "phytonutrient" is an unfortunate choice of terminology. Substances such as the isoflavones in soy (e.g., genistein and daidzein) and the lignans (e.g., enterolactone) in flaxseed, as well as the products derived from them, are *not* estrogens, but their *similarity* to estrogens allows them to *block* excess estrogens, perhaps preventing their negative effects. Germs living in a healthy intestine convert isoflavones and lignans into messenger molecules called equol and enterolactone that modulate hormone chemistry and affect cell division and the growth of blood vessels. The higher your level of equol and enterolactone, the lower is your risk for reproductive cancer.

23:00
24:00
25:00
01:00
02:00
03:00
04:00
05:00
06:00
07:00
08:00
09:00
10:00
11:00
12:00
13:00
14:00
15:00
16:00
17:00

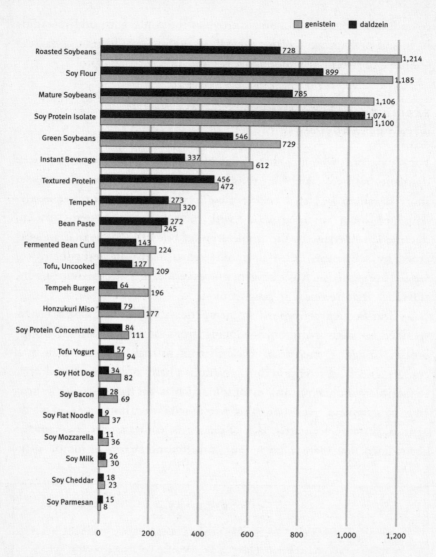

Isoflavone content of soy foods. The figures in this chart for genistein and daidzein (the two main isoflavones) are in micrograms per gram. These are rough estimates; the content of these substances in any given soy product depends on the way the soybeans are grown and processed. Soy, flaxseed, and rye fiber have been proven to best promote healthy hormone chemistry and reduce your risk factors. They are convenient and potent. But for more variety, or if you cannot tolerate soy or flaxseed, other readily available foods that are rich in isoflavones and lignans include seeds (particularly rapeseed and sunflower), whole legumes, legume sprouts (including soybeans, fava beans, mung beans, Adzuki beans, and alfalfa), whole grains, berries, dried seaweeds, vegetables, and fruits.

nancy, or other condition—that can be registered in a standard laboratory test. Unfortunately, this situation often leads a woman to feel that she's a victim of her body's glands. Men with chronic prostate problems frequently feel similarly victimized.

The simple measure of adding soy and flaxseed to the diet will help many people who suffer from such "hormone problems."

PHYTONUTRIENTS AND THE RHYTHM OF LIFE

As researchers continue to unravel the costs of ignoring phytonutrients in food, there will be a scientifically based return to eating in ways that will more effectively synchronize your body's rhythm with the natural flow of time. I believe that this approach to diet will be grounded on the understanding of how certain food substances serve as seasonal indicators for animals. It may turn out that seasonal changes in food consumption are also important for humans; what we know already is that certain phytonutrients have a salutary effect on the human reproductive system and other important aspects of health whenever they are consumed.

Whether or not you have "hormone problems," developing the habit of consuming foods rich in phytonutrients is also worthwhile for the long-term protection they offer against more serious illnesses. Already, researchers have evidence that these plant-derived substances have effects that go beyond the reproductive system. For example, studies have shown that soy lowers cholesterol, reduces the risk of cardiovascular disease, provides antioxidant protection, and helps prevent osteoporosis.[3]

The daily consumption of soy protein, flaxseed, and other phytonutrient sources is a key element of the Circadian Diet, because the long-term benefits of doing so are so important. Since the phytonutrients in plants enhance the capacity of animals to live in synchrony with time, it simply makes sense that consuming phytonutrient-rich foods every day enhances your body's rhythmic functioning. You can take pleasure in knowing that beneath this approach is your participation in a fundamental rule of nature: Living things exist in time.

24:00
25:00
01:00
02:00
03:00
04:00
05:00
06:00
07:00
08:00
09:00
10:00
11:00
12:00
13:00
14:00
15:00
16:00
17:00
18:00
19:00
20:00
21:00
22:00
23:00
24:00
25:00
01:00

CHAPTER

4

Carbohydrates: Life Is Sweet

Luke Imperiale runs heavy equipment. Luke himself is heavy equipment. Big hands, big face, big body, big belly, big heart. Big problems. Until he retired last year at age sixty-five, he had never missed a day at work. But he admits that he never felt good, either. He just worked, enduring his feelings of fatigue, anxiety, and depression along with constant digestive problems, persistent rashes, and fungal skin infections, and a host of other complaints. Luke had made the rounds of all the specialists. Although the list of medications he was taking required graph paper to keep it all straight, he still felt miserable.

He started feeling better after I helped him bring his food allergies and fungal infections under control, but he was still suffering from episodes of what he called "the shakes." Luke's diet was all carbohydrates—lots of sandwiches and donuts and, because he loved it, bread at every meal. He had an afternoon candy bar habit, which he indulged even though it always made him sleepy.

What made him turn the corner, leaving him feeling well and ending "the shakes," was moderating his enormous consumption of carbohydrates and moving it into the evening. Today, he has most of his carbohydrates at supper. He drinks a protein shake or eats protein, like a turkey patty or piece of chicken, for breakfast. At lunch he has a salad with chicken, some baked ham, or a piece of fish or meat. When he wants a snack, he eats nuts instead of donuts. And at dinner he has fish or meat, vegetables, and his beloved bread.

The change in his overall health and vitality has been enormous. "All I'm doing is moving my food around and drinking the protein shake, which tastes like ice cream. It's made a one hundred percent difference in how I feel," says Luke. "I have a tremendous amount of energy, and even my outlook on life is different. I don't have that low feeling or anxiety. I used to get up tired every morning. Now I do things around the house, where I didn't have the desire before. And my digestion is great; I don't get that blown up, bloated feeling any more."

Luke had a complicated story, and it would not do justice to him or to his problems to try to put it all under one heading. But one theme emerges from his story that is relevant to all of us—a carbohydrate-heavy diet.

CARBOHYDRATES ARE CONCENTRATED SUNLIGHT

In the 1800s when scientists first focused on the goodness, or what we today call nutritional value, in foods, they determined that there were three main components: carbohydrates, protein, and fats. Today, if you take all the edible material at the average supermarket, you will find that most of it, by weight, is composed of carbohydrates. Picture foods like bananas, a bowl of rice, bread, potatoes, pasta, and just about any snack food; if a food is white, and it's not a milk product or egg white, it's made mostly of carbohydrate. And if it is sweet to the taste, unless it contains some artificial sweetener, it is carbohydrate. Anything of vegetable origin—that is, it starts out as a plant growing in or on the earth—ends up being carbohydrate in your diet.

There are two exceptions to this rule that fall into the protein category: the bean family, particularly soybeans, and a certain type of blue-green algae, called spirulina, that has entered the food supply in the form of a supplement. (For lists of foods and a breakdown of their carbohydrate, protein, fat, calories, and other nutrients, see the charts at the end of this chapter.)

From the earliest times, because people burned oil and woody plants for heat and light, they grasped the connection between these fuels on the one hand and heat and light, on the other. More than a hundred years ago scientists recognized that the process of producing heat and light was going on in humans and other living beings. This metabolic fire does not actually produce visible light, but it does involve the release within the body of "sunlight." That's because carbohydrate is concentrated sunlight. Green plants capture sunlight in one of the most fundamental processes of biochemistry, called photosynthesis. The sun's energy joins carbon dioxide (*carbo*) in the air with water (*hydrate*) to form carbohydrates, whose molecules are joined end to end in one of two different ways, as starches or as cellulose.

Starches are the digestible part of plant foods, releasing sugars when they are broken down. But not all carbohydrates are easily broken down into sugars. Although the basic units of all carbohydrates are sugar molecules (glucose and fructose), cellulose—the indigestible, woody, fibrous part of plants, sometimes called dietary fiber—has a different chemical structure from digestible carbohydrates.

Animals that consume leaves, sticks, and other woody parts of plants can digest the cellulose only because they have cellulose-digesting germs in their intestines, just like those that are in the soil and that help sticks and leaves decay. Human beings are different; you cannot usefully eat a matchstick. Your intestinal germs do not use their capacity to digest cellulose to serve you energy; instead, they eat the cellulose and serve you in other ways, releasing from the fiber necessary molecules that you can't make for yourself.

You eat starchy and sugary carbohydrates to recover the sun's energy, captured in the plants that supply your food. There is a vast array of carbohydrate-containing foods. Unprocessed plant foods give you digestible sugars and starches and indigestible (but important) cellulose. These include tubers, like potato; roots, such as rutabaga, sweet potato, beet, turnip, carrot, parsnip, and cassava; seeds, like rice, wheat, oats, barley, corn, millet, buckwheat, nuts, and beans; leaves, such as lettuce and other greens; as well as other foods that come from the stems, fruits, and flowers of plants. Processing of certain starchy plant foods yields corn starch, potato starch, and starch that's made from rice. These foods may seem different, but their starches all consist of long chains of small sugar molecules joined end to end to form huge molecules. And you digest them all in more or less the same way.

Although various carbohydrates—a mouthful of rice, an apple, and a matchstick, for example—do not appear to be equally moist, their molecules all have the same water content. When you burn the match it releases heat as well as water and carbon dioxide in the rising smoke; this process is the transformation of the carbohydrates of the match back into air and light. The same thing happens to the rice, apple, or other carbohydrates you eat. Between your dinner plate and your bloodstream, your digestive tract breaks starchy carbohydrates down into simple sugar molecules. Then these molecules move through your bloodstream and, with the help of a hormone called insulin, into your body's cells, where they are burned as fuel. When you burn carbohydrates in your body's metabolic fire, you exhale carbon dioxide and water in your breath; just like the smoke from the burning match, your metabolic smoke is restoring the basic ingredients of carbohydrates (carbon dioxide and water) to the air they came from. But your body conserves the heat from the fire of apple or rice so that it can become the energy that drives your physical and mental activities.

This process of taking sugar molecules apart to extract their energy is essentially the same for all living things. It is also the same basic process involved in any kind of burning. There are a few exceptions, the most notable being the combustion of oils.

CARBOHYDRATES PROVIDE ENERGY FOR YOUR BODY'S NIGHTTIME TASKS

High carbohydrate foods, then, provide a rich source of quick energy and heat. And circadian rhythm dictates that the time when you most need them is at night.[1] Most people have it backwards, believing that you need carbohydrates for daytime energy and not so much at night, when you are resting. But you're not really resting. While your muscles and brain do slow down in their use of energy at night, your whole body is doing healing and repair work, and your liver is involved in detoxification. In fact, one of the key reasons you sleep at night is that your body is so engaged with energy-consuming chores that it doesn't have enough resources to keep consciousness, biochemical replenishment, and detoxification all going at once.

Carbohydrates provide the large amount of fuel your body requires overnight for synthesis, or the making of new molecules. First, the molecules that you use up during the day, when you are active, must be repaired and replaced. Second, toxins and other substances, like burned-out hormones and neurotransmitters, must be disposed of. Generally, when you rid your body of unwanted substances, you can't just throw them away. Although it sounds strange, you have to synthesize new molecules in order to safely remove the worn-out ones. Your body must first package each molecule and provide a vehicle to take it away. Your metabolic budget for bagging the waste and carting it away is more than you spend on any other activity because your sanitation department visits and serves every other department in your body.

The liver is in charge of this disposal process; it also makes and supplies molecules for other organs. The liver does its heaviest work on the night shift. As the sun goes down, the lights go on in the liver, and this supremely important factory of the body has until dawn to finish many of its biochemical chores. The liver sustains a significant weight loss in the process, most of which is accounted for by a drop in glycogen. At bedtime about 15 percent of your liver's weight is glycogen, an animal starch your body draws on to keep your blood sugar up at night. By morning, glycogen stores are reduced to about 1 percent of the liver's weight. The factory metaphor is apt because the synthesis of new molecules is much like an assembly line where large, complex products are made out of small, simple parts in a predetermined sequence. Sequencing underlies the wonderful efficiency that your body brings to all its tasks.

You might wonder why you can go all night without eating when if you did the same thing during the day, you'd become hungry. While you sleep, when your muscles and brain consume less energy, and the rest of your body is engaged in repair, healing, and detoxification, your body maintains a high level of sugar in the blood.[2] The sustained sweetness of your blood at night is your body's way of delivering the sun's energy to your liver and all the other organs.

During the day your body sustains a lower blood sugar level that keeps tumbling down unless you eat. Let's say you eat a certain amount of carbohydrates at 8:00 a.m. and then go without food for the next eight hours.

Those breakfast carbohydrates, regardless of your activity, will get used up, and your blood sugar will fall long before that energy is needed during the night. Your body manages your evening carbohydrates differently. When you eat the same amount of carbohydrates in the evening, your body is able to keep a uniform blood sugar level between the hours of midnight and 6:00 a.m. by converting glycogen to glucose, even though you are not eating anything. Without an evening load of carbohydrates, though, your body will have a harder time keeping your blood sweet.

CARBOHYDRATES AND SLEEP

The Circadian Diet often relieves poor sleep, which is a common complaint. In a survey done by the National Sleep Foundation in 1998 and 1999, more than 60 percent of American adults reported having sleep-related problems at least a few nights a week. The most obvious effects are traffic accidents—sleepy drivers are responsible for more than one hundred thousand police-reported crashes per year—and daytime drowsiness that decreases alertness, causes difficulty in concentration, and interferes with daily activities. In the same survey, 40 percent of American adults reported being so sleepy during the day that it interfered with their daily activities.[3]

But the effects of poor sleep can be far more subtle. Sleep loss is associated with depressed mood and altered hormone production. Some research has shown that even one night's sleep loss weakens the immune system, lessening the body's ability to fight off colds, flu, and other infections.[4] And Italian researchers at the University of Pavia believe that sleep deprivation is linked to heart attacks and strokes the next morning.[5]

If you put off consuming carbohydrates until evening, you will sleep better. Not only are you providing your body with the appropriate raw materials it needs to do its nighttime work, but the carbohydrates also allow the absorption of tryptophan and other nutrients that are needed for sleep. Carbohydrates are like the ferryboat that tryptophan uses to cross the river to your brain, where it is converted to serotonin, the mother of the family of nighttime neurotransmitters.

TOO MANY CARBOHYDRATES AND INSULIN RESISTANCE

On the other hand, even though carbohydrates are an essential source of energy and a boon to healthy sleep, you can get too much of a good thing. On average, Americans consume nearly 52 percent of their calories in carbohydrates, many of them starchy and sugary.[6] This is a relatively recent phenomenon in human history, and it's the root of a number of serious health ailments. Problems with carbohydrate metabolism and specifically a disorder called hyperinsulinism, Syndrome X, or insulin resistance underlie many conditions that have been traditionally blamed on high cholesterol.

If you were to go back in your family and count four generations for every one hundred years, forty generations would take you back to the

23:00
24:00
25:00
01:00
02:00
03:00
04:00
05:00
06:00
07:00
08:00
09:00
10:00
11:00
12:00
13:00
14:00
15:00
16:00
17:00
18:00
19:00
20:00
21:00
22:00
23:00
24:00
25:00
01:00
02:00
03:00
04:00
05:00
06:00
07:00
08:00

SYNDROME X: CARBOHYDRATE POISONING

- In the dark night kitchen, a woman stands bathed in the refrigerator light. She has come there to relieve her insomnia by getting a snack.

- A red-faced man with some private urgency moves desperately past you in line, pushing you and his neighbors with his enormous belly. People move aside, but it's not because of his size. He looks as if he is going to not just pop his buttons but actually explode.

- An adult woman endures the return of a kind of adolescence from hell in which her body changes again. But this time she has acne that threatens to be permanent, hair growing in undesired places, and a change in her body from shapely to shapeless as the inches increase on her abdomen instead of her chest.

These are three faces of Syndrome X, named in 1988 by Dr. Gerald M. Reaven, to acknowledge a cluster of symptoms that, even more than most conditions, resisted description as a "disease entity."

Syndrome X is a variable cluster of symptoms with one underlying feature: a poor attachment of insulin to the cells for which it is the usher for glucose. Glucose passes from the bloodstream to be used for energy inside cells only when insulin is able to deliver it. The inefficiency of insulin which, in its extreme form, year 1000, and four hundred generations would date back ten thousand years. Your four hundred–times great-grandparents were just like you, except for what you might call lifestyle. In terms of their genetic makeup, intelligence, emotions, basic needs for food, shelter, and getting along with others, and particularly their nutritional requirements, they were so much like you that one of their babies dropped into your family would be no different from the other children of your family.

You can be quite certain that your four hundred–times great-grandparents spent most of their time looking for food. Not only did they not have a supermarket, they did not even have farms. Every day, or as often as they could, they went out searching for food wherever they happened to be. They and their ancestors had been gathering food from the environment since the beginning of time. Humans have been eating the

---

is the hallmark of late onset diabetes, makes the body adapt by escalating insulin levels so that more glucose will get taken to its destination.

Insulin has other jobs besides ushering glucose, so when insulin levels rise, a number of undesirable things happen, affecting the capacity of cells to burn sugar efficiently, make message-carrying molecules (informational substances), and mobilize and synthesize fat. In the pre- or nondiabetic person, the extra insulin impairs the body's normal ability to sustain blood sugar during the night, triggering nighttime trips from bedroom to kitchen. In addition, the high levels of insulin act upon the metabolism of the steroid hormones that come from the adrenal glands and the sex glands, resulting in hypertension, obesity, and difficulty with weight loss. Extra pounds are typically found around the middle of the body. Women with Syndrome X also suffer from abnormal hair growth and acne.

Even without changing the amount of fiber or protein in the diet, people with Syndrome X or Type II diabetes can bring their insulin levels down by increasing dietary fat from 30 to 45 percent and cutting carbohydrates from 55 to 45 percent. But you can do much better by following the Circadian Diet, going very lightly on carbohydrates in the morning and noon meals and emphasizing foods with a low glycemic index. These foods produce a much lower rise in blood glucose and insulin following eating than do similar foods with the same caloric value. Low glycemic index foods include beans, basmati rice, barley, and vegetables that are low in starch. Increasing the fiber content of your diet is especially helpful.

products of agriculture such as cereal grains and milk from domesticated animals for a very small part of our history. When we talk about a "normal" diet it's important to define what that means, especially when it comes to carbohydrates. What do you suppose, taking the long view, is a normal diet for human beings? I'm not suggesting that you go back to eating the diet of a cave person. But one of the central points of this book is that normal food intake for most of our human history did not include many starchy and sugary carbohydrates. The food gathering you do in the supermarket gives you easier access to much larger quantities—and far worse quality—of carbohydrates than were ever available to your distant ancestors.

Think about it. If you go into the woods outside of town on a given day and try to find food for dinner, you're not going to find many edible carbohydrates in the natural environment unless you come across somebody's farm. You'll probably discover some nuts, berries, and small fruits, but only when they're in season. The bulk of your dinner will be made up of whatever creatures you can catch, which means that your diet will have a substantial share of protein and fat but relatively little in the way of starches. And the carbohydrates that you consume will have, like your ancestors' diet, ten times more fiber than those in your current diet.

Now let's go back to your four hundred–times great-grandmother. She's out there one day looking for food, and she comes across a bunch of sweet berries. She has no way to put these up into jars of jelly; instead, she has to exploit the berry patch while it's in season by eating the fruit on the spot or taking it home. If she is blessed with an evolutionary advantage and her body has a knack for exploiting this sudden surprise of available carbohydrates, she will be able to use some of it as an immediate source of energy and store the rest as fat for later use. The knack she has involves raising her serum insulin level quickly.

Here's what the insulin does. Throughout all of nature, life takes place in the cells of the body. Your body consists of about one hundred trillion cells. Approximately two-thirds of the water inside of your body is inside these cells; it's called intracellular fluid. In between the cells and bathing them is another kind of water, called extracellular fluid. Your bloodstream contains a mixture of the two in the form of serum and red and white cells.

The one hundred trillion cells of your body require sugar as a source of energy. Glucose, the sugar that comes from the breakdown of carbohydrate-containing foods, travels through the bloodstream into the fluid around the cells. When it arrives, it requires a special carrier to get it into the cells, just like an old-fashioned locomotive needed a fireman to shovel the coal from the coal bin into the engine. That carrier is insulin. Once inside, the glucose is transferred deep inside the cell to other compartments, called the mitochondria, where it is burned to provide energy.

In your ancestors' time, carbohydrate loads were few and far between—they certainly didn't occur more often than once a day. So the ability to raise serum insulin levels in response to the carbohydrates as soon as they came on board was a plus; it was adaptive. It helped people store extra carbohydrates as fat, and the fatter they were, the more resistant to famine they became, allowing them and their offspring to survive. This evolutionary advantage is why people with this trait were your four hundred–times great-grandparents; people without the knack to raise serum insulin levels tended not to make it.

Many of us inherited from our food-gathering ancestors this capacity for raising serum insulin levels when exposed to carbohydrates. If you can accept the fact that your body's chemistry is geared for the relatively infrequent and sparse intake of carbohydrates, you may wonder what happens when you shift gears into modern times. You now have an essentially endless supply of carbohydrates, and you can consume them frequently. When your inherited ability to respond by jacking up your serum insulin levels is triggered this frequently, there are undesirable consequences.

Insulin levels rise in response to quantity of carbohydrate intake, and they escalate in response to frequent carbohydrate intake. For example, if you eat a big bowl of pasta and a banana split, your body must produce a significant amount of insulin in order to convert the derived sugars into energy and fat. If you then stay away from a carbohydrate load, your insulin level will reset to a normal, healthy figure. If, however, you consume sweet and starchy foods several times a day, each consumption will bump up your insulin level so it becomes ratcheted to a persistently and undesirably high level.

In some people this escalation is more pronounced and leads to insulin resistance, which can be a path to Type II diabetes. (Type I, or childhood onset diabetes, is associated with insulin deficiency, as opposed to Type II, or late onset diabetes, in which there is excessive, ineffective, and harmful insulin.) Many more people have insulin resistance than are diabetic, but the two problems overlap to a considerable degree. Insulin resistance is a significant contributing factor to cardiovascular disease, diabetes, chronic inflammatory problems such as colitis, arthritis, and asthma, and disturbances of mood and behavior.

If you score high on the Insulin Resistance checklist, the Circadian Diet will curb the tendency to raise your serum insulin levels because you'll be eating carbohydrates less frequently. You don't have to severely cut back the quantity of carbohydrates you eat unless you want to restrict calories to lose weight. Instead, I'm suggesting that you limit how often you eat carbohydrates so that you don't repeatedly push up your serum insulin levels, putting yourself at risk from the harmful consequences just mentioned. Less frequently means eating the bulk of your starchy and sugary food once a day. And as you've already learned, the time of day when your body most needs the fuel provided by carbohydrates is evening, to prepare for its heavy night work of detoxification, repair, restoration, and providing heat.

Whether or not you suffer from insulin resistance, eating in accordance with Nature's plan—your circadian rhythm—is beneficial for you. As long as you put off most of your carbohydrate intake until evening, it's not harmful to eat protein at dinner. But you should consume most of your protein at breakfast and lunch, as I'll explain in the next chapter.

INSULIN RESISTANCE CHECKLIST

Score yourself by entering a 0 for NONE, 1 for MILD, 2 for MODERATE, and 3 for SEVERE

		Score
Weight, appetite, and food:		
Difficulty losing weight		
Waist bigger than hips (apple obesity)		
Sugar craving		
Salt sensitivity (water retention)		
Skin and hair:		
Hair grows where you don't want it		
Hair thins where you do want it		
Acne now		
Other conditions:		
Polycystic ovaries		
High blood pressure		
Chronic fungal infection		
Kidney stones (calcium oxalate)		
Family history:		
Diabetes (adult onset)		
Heart disease		
High blood pressure		
Body chemistry:		
High blood triglycerides	Add 2	
Low HDL (high density lipoproteins)	Add 2	
Abnormal "liver function tests"	Add 2	
Increased serum uric acid	Add 2	
Low serum magnesium	Add 2	
Increased serum ferritin	Add 2	
Total score		

Maximum score is 54

Minimum score is 0

Less than 10 is good

10–19 is fair

Above 20 is poor

If you have any of the following, you have insulin resistance by definition:

- Type II Diabetes (adult onset)
- High serum insulin
- Hyperinsulinemic glucose tolerance test
- Borderline hemoglobin A1c (6.4-7)

Use this checklist to determine if you have a tendency toward high serum insulin levels.

CALORIC CONTENT AND COMPOSITION OF BREAKFAST FOODS

This list is sorted with the highest percent carbohydrate food at the top. Each bar, which is sized proportionately for the number of calories per food, shows the percentage of total calories for starch, protein, sugar, fiber, fat, and saturated fat. Labels on the left show the food, the number of calories per serving, and the serving size. The number appearing under the bars are grams per serving.

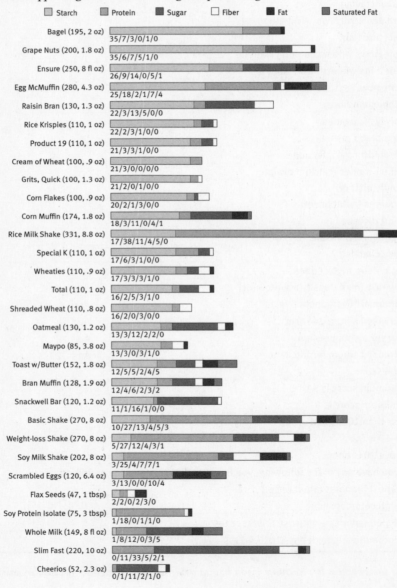

| | Starch | Protein | Sugar | Fiber | Fat | Saturated Fat |

Bagel (195, 2 oz)
35/7/3/0/1/0

Grape Nuts (200, 1.8 oz)
35/6/7/5/1/0

Ensure (250, 8 fl oz)
26/9/14/0/5/1

Egg McMuffin (280, 4.3 oz)
25/18/2/1/7/4

Raisin Bran (130, 1.3 oz)
22/3/13/5/0/0

Rice Krispies (110, 1 oz)
22/2/3/1/0/0

Product 19 (110, 1 oz)
21/3/3/1/0/0

Cream of Wheat (100, .9 oz)
21/3/0/0/0/0

Grits, Quick (100, 1.3 oz)
21/2/0/1/0/0

Corn Flakes (100, .9 oz)
20/2/1/3/0/0

Corn Muffin (174, 1.8 oz)
18/3/11/0/4/1

Rice Milk Shake (331, 8.8 oz)
17/38/11/4/5/0

Special K (110, 1 oz)
17/6/3/1/0/0

Wheaties (110, .9 oz)
17/3/3/3/1/0

Total (110, 1 oz)
16/2/5/3/1/0

Shreaded Wheat (110, .8 oz)
16/2/0/3/0/0

Oatmeal (130, 1.2 oz)
13/3/12/2/2/0

Maypo (85, 3.8 oz)
13/3/0/3/1/0

Toast w/Butter (152, 1.8 oz)
12/5/5/2/4/5

Bran Muffin (128, 1.9 oz)
12/4/6/2/3/2

Snackwell Bar (120, 1.2 oz)
11/1/16/1/0/0

Basic Shake (270, 8 oz)
10/27/13/4/5/3

Weight-loss Shake (270, 8 oz)
5/27/12/4/3/1

Soy Milk Shake (202, 8 oz)
3/25/4/7/7/1

Scrambled Eggs (120, 6.4 oz)
3/13/0/0/10/4

Flax Seeds (47, 1 tbsp)
2/2/0/2/3/0

Soy Protein Isolate (75, 3 tbsp)
1/18/0/1/1/0

Whole Milk (149, 8 fl oz)
1/8/12/0/3/5

Slim Fast (220, 10 oz)
0/11/33/5/2/1

Cheerios (52, 2.3 oz)
0/1/11/2/1/0

CALORIC CONTENT AND COMPOSITION OF LUNCH FOODS

This list is sorted with the highest percent carbohydrate foods at the top. Each bar, which is sized proportionately for the number of calories per food, shows the percentage of total calories for starch, protein, sugar, fiber, fat, and saturated fat. Labels on the left show the food, the number of calories per serving, and the serving size. The numbers appearing under the bars are grams per serving.

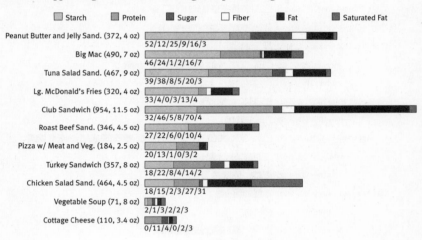

CALORIC CONTENT AND COMPOSITION OF SNACK FOODS

This list is sorted with the highest percent carbohydrate foods at the top. Each bar, which is sized proportionately for the number of calories per food, shows the percentage of total calories for starch, protein, sugar, fiber, fat, and saturated fat. Labels on the left show the food, the number of calories per serving, and the serving size. The numbers appearing under the bars are grams per serving.

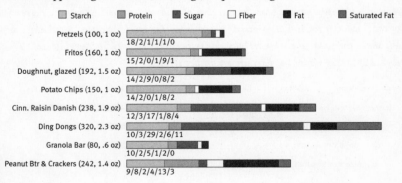

(cont'd)

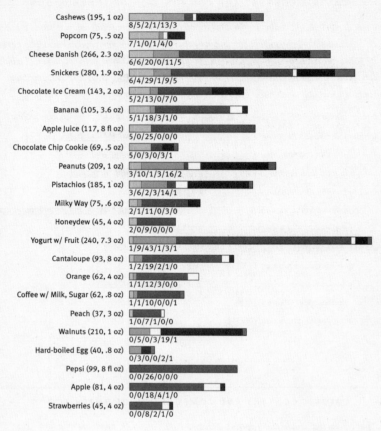

Cashews (195, 1 oz) — 8/5/2/1/13/3
Popcorn (75, .5 oz) — 7/1/0/1/4/0
Cheese Danish (266, 2.3 oz) — 6/6/20/0/11/5
Snickers (280, 1.9 oz) — 6/4/29/1/9/5
Chocolate Ice Cream (143, 2 oz) — 5/2/13/0/7/0
Banana (105, 3.6 oz) — 5/1/18/3/1/0
Apple Juice (117, 8 fl oz) — 5/0/25/0/0/0
Chocolate Chip Cookie (69, .5 oz) — 5/0/3/0/3/1
Peanuts (209, 1 oz) — 3/10/1/3/16/2
Pistachios (185, 1 oz) — 3/6/2/3/14/1
Milky Way (75, .6 oz) — 2/1/11/0/3/0
Honeydew (45, 4 oz) — 2/0/9/0/0/0
Yogurt w/ Fruit (240, 7.3 oz) — 1/9/43/1/3/1
Cantaloupe (93, 8 oz) — 1/2/19/2/1/0
Orange (62, 4 oz) — 1/1/12/3/0/0
Coffee w/ Milk, Sugar (62, .8 oz) — 1/1/10/0/0/1
Peach (37, 3 oz) — 1/0/7/1/0/0
Walnuts (210, 1 oz) — 0/5/0/3/19/1
Hard-boiled Egg (40, .8 oz) — 0/3/0/0/2/1
Pepsi (99, 8 fl oz) — 0/0/26/0/0/0
Apple (81, 4 oz) — 0/0/18/4/1/0
Strawberries (45, 4 oz) — 0/0/8/2/1/0

CALORIC CONTENT AND COMPOSITION OF DINNER FOODS

This list is sorted with the highest percent carbohydrate foods at the top. Each bar, which is sized proportionately for the number of calories per food, shows the percentage of total calories for starch, protein, sugar, fiber, fat, and saturated fat. Labels on the left show the food, the number of calories per serving, and the serving size. The numbers appearing under the bars are grams per serving.

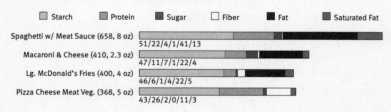

☐ Starch   ☐ Protein   ☐ Sugar   ☐ Fiber   ☐ Fat   ☐ Saturated Fat

Spaghetti w/ Meat Sauce (658, 8 oz) — 51/22/4/1/41/13
Macaroni & Cheese (410, 2.3 oz) — 47/11/7/1/22/4
Lg. McDonald's Fries (400, 4 oz) — 46/6/1/4/22/5
Pizza Cheese Meat Veg. (368, 5 oz) — 43/26/2/0/11/3

(cont'd)

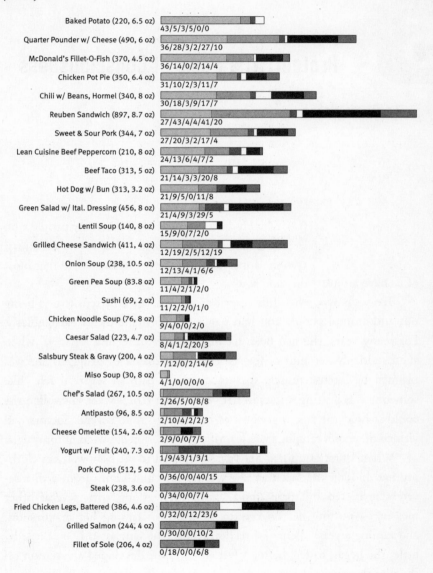

Food	Values
Baked Potato (220, 6.5 oz)	43/5/3/5/0/0
Quarter Pounder w/ Cheese (490, 6 oz)	36/28/3/2/27/10
McDonald's Fillet-O-Fish (370, 4.5 oz)	36/14/0/2/14/4
Chicken Pot Pie (350, 6.4 oz)	31/10/2/3/11/7
Chili w/ Beans, Hormel (340, 8 oz)	30/18/3/9/17/7
Reuben Sandwich (897, 8.7 oz)	27/43/4/4/41/20
Sweet & Sour Pork (344, 7 oz)	27/20/3/2/17/4
Lean Cuisine Beef Peppercorn (210, 8 oz)	24/13/6/4/7/2
Beef Taco (313, 5 oz)	21/14/3/3/20/8
Hot Dog w/ Bun (313, 3.2 oz)	21/9/5/0/11/8
Green Salad w/ Ital. Dressing (456, 8 oz)	21/4/9/3/29/5
Lentil Soup (140, 8 oz)	15/9/0/7/2/0
Grilled Cheese Sandwich (411, 4 oz)	12/19/2/5/12/19
Onion Soup (238, 10.5 oz)	12/13/4/1/6/6
Green Pea Soup (83.8 oz)	11/4/2/1/2/0
Sushi (69, 2 oz)	11/2/2/0/1/0
Chicken Noodle Soup (76, 8 oz)	9/4/0/0/2/0
Caesar Salad (223, 4.7 oz)	8/4/1/2/20/3
Salsbury Steak & Gravy (200, 4 oz)	7/12/0/2/14/6
Miso Soup (30, 8 oz)	4/1/0/0/0/0
Chef's Salad (267, 10.5 oz)	2/26/5/0/8/8
Antipasto (96, 8.5 oz)	2/10/4/2/2/3
Cheese Omelette (154, 2.6 oz)	2/9/0/0/7/5
Yogurt w/ Fruit (240, 7.3 oz)	1/9/43/1/3/1
Pork Chops (512, 5 oz)	0/36/0/0/40/15
Steak (238, 3.6 oz)	0/34/0/0/7/4
Fried Chicken Legs, Battered (386, 4.6 oz)	0/32/0/12/23/6
Grilled Salmon (244, 4 oz)	0/30/0/0/10/2
Fillet of Sole (206, 4 oz)	0/18/0/0/6/8

24:00
25:00
01:00
02:00
03:00
04:00
05:00
06:00
07:00
08:00
09:00
10:00
11:00
12:00
13:00
14:00
15:00
16:00
17:00
18:00
19:00
20:00
21:00
22:00
23:00
24:00
25:00
01:00

CHAPTER

5

Protein: The Basis of Consciousness

Leslie Hudson is a survivor. Like many people who have endured abuse and other forms of injury, she appears to lack the protective shield that most of us have around body and soul.

Ten years ago, when I first saw her, she was fearfully sensitive to being out and around people and had panic attacks if she didn't eat regularly. For many years, she had been having episodes of feeling "spacey," when she'd suddenly get faint or feel as if she were drunk or drugged. She was plagued by intense muscle spasms and joint pain so severe it felt "like someone was putting knives in her veins." Her hands were so swollen she couldn't hold the steering wheel of her car. Visits to several doctors had yielded diagnoses ranging from arthritis to borderline lupus to fibromyalgia.

When I first examined her I was surprised to see how well her clothing had hidden the fact that she was all skin and bones from a diet severely restricted by many food sensitivities. Along with several other measures—putting her on certain vitamins, increasing her magnesium, and taming a yeast allergy—I recommended the Circadian Diet. Little by little, she began to feel better. Over time, Leslie developed a variation on the diet that worked best for her. These days, she eats a small amount of protein at breakfast but has the bulk of her protein, and her main meal of the day, at noon; she eats no protein at night. As a result, she says, "my energy has increased one thousand percent and I am so steady. I feel better now than I have for twenty-five or thirty years."

Leslie's response was unusual because she was already on a fairly high protein diet before she added carbohydrates to her evening meal and concentrated her protein during the day as I recommended. However, most people notice the benefits of restricting carbohydrates in the daytime more than the results of adding carbohydrates or avoiding protein in the evening.

PROTEIN IN THE BODY

How could such a simple change in Leslie's diet make such a big difference? And what exactly is protein?

While the structure of carbohydrate, or starch, is simple, that of protein is complex. Starch is made of big molecules that are composed of the same little molecule joined over and over to itself like a paper clip chain made from just two different boxes of paper clips. Protein is like a chain made from twenty boxes of paper clips of varying sizes and shapes.

There are estimated to be thirty-thousand distinct proteins in the body. The difference from one to another depends on the number and sequence of the "paper clips"—or amino acids—that make up the protein. The chain of amino acids is arranged like a spiral that folds upon itself, producing a variety of shapes. Long, fibrous proteins are found in hair and skin (keratin) and connective tissue (collagen); they are the basic structural materials of your body. Globular proteins like hemoglobin, the red material in blood, have specialized functions as carriers. Other proteins, such as antibodies, take on specific shapes to serve as labels the immune system uses to remember and identify everything it encounters. The proteins called enzymes are big, shapely molecules whose embrace is essential to assembling or disconnecting all the small molecules in the body's chemical economy.

Protein from food is essential to the growth and maintenance of all body tissues. You can live without carbohydrates in your diet, but without protein you'd die, after becoming dull, irritable, and listless. I saw this happen when I worked in parts of Africa where babies are weaned from mother's milk to a white, starchy gruel. After a few months on this protein-free sustenance, they became inconsolably cranky, pale, puffy, and swollen. Without careful reintroduction of protein foods, they died. It is a long way from Africa and this disease, called kwashiorkor, to the United States and a condition that makes many people cranky, spacey, puffy, and pale. But the feel of the two conditions is similar and has to do with related disturbances in the dietary balance between protein and carbohydrate.

NITROGEN MAKES THE DIFFERENCE

What distinguishes the amino acids that make up protein from the sugars that compose carbohydrate is nitrogen. Remember, carbohydrate is made out of air, sunlight, and water. If you have no background in biochemistry this may sound a little fanciful because air—or, in this case, carbon dioxide, which makes up one-twentieth of the air we breathe—combined with water and sunlight don't sound very substantial. But that's just what carbohydrate is.

Protein also begins in the air. Take a deep breath. Eighty percent of what you're breathing is nitrogen; it makes up most of the earth's atmosphere. Our planet is blanketed with a protective layer of nitrogen fifty miles thick. Nitrogen is tasteless, odorless, and relatively inert, meaning that it doesn't combine easily with other substances. Otherwise, it wouldn't be good material for making an atmosphere, which needs to bathe all of the things that live on earth but not mix with them.

But in the world of chemistry it's not unusual for the personality of a pure element to change when it is combined with others. For example, ordinary table salt is made of two elements—sodium and chlorine—that are deadly poisons in their elementary forms but viable in their combined state. When nitrogen joins carbon dioxide and water, it forms protein molecules with a variety of sizes and intricate shapes, diverse functions, and many differences in texture, taste, and color.

The carbohydrates on our planet are more or less the same from one kind of living being to another. The nitrogen-based proteins, on the other hand, are different from one organism to another even though there may be some common themes in terms of shape, size, and complexity. So much do they differ that proteins may not be compatible when taken from one creature into another. That's why transplanted organs are bound to be

PROTEINS AND ALLERGY

Your body contains three kinds of information-carrying molecules. Your chromosomes and genes are made of DNA, which carries information from your ancestors about how to be you. Proteins are another kind of information-carrying molecule. Their information is the basis for the way that different parts of you (your liver, kidneys, and so on) perform their functions. Finally, your body makes other small molecules that carry information from one part of you to another; these include steroid hormones, prostaglandin hormones, neuropeptides, cytokines, lymphokines and endorphins; collectively they can be called informational substances.

Many of your body's informational substances are peptides, short chains of amino acids. Amino acids, you recall, are the "paper clips" that in much longer chains, form proteins. You make these peptides to carry messages. Some, called neuropeptides, carry messages in your nervous system to regulate perception of pain, mood, attention, and other cognitive functions. Other peptides carry out activities in the immune, endocrine, digestive, and other systems. The protein you eat plays a critical role in providing the raw materials for this communication system.

But sometimes a problem develops during the breakdown of the proteins you eat. These proteins are digested by undoing the connections between the paper clips that compose them. For at least a time during digestion, short chains of paper clips—two, three, up to a dozen or more—are released. These short chains are also peptides, and they may enter your bloodstream without further digestion. Although this can happen in healthy people, it is more likely to occur in a person whose digestive tract has been made more permeable by illness or injury.

These peptides, which have come from your food, may so closely resemble the peptides in your own communication system that they become false messengers when they enter the bloodstream. While this probably happens with peptides from a variety of foods, those that have been most closely studied are cereal grains such as wheat, rye, and barley, in which "gluten" is the name of the protein whose digestion liberates undesirable peptides. In addition, milk from any animal can yield peptides from a protein called casein. These false messengers from peptides can cause serious consequences. For example, a team of researchers led by Alan Friedman at Johnson and Johnson's Ortho Division in Rochester, New York, have identified peptides liberated from casein in the urine of autistic children that are identical to the hallucinogen found in the toxins of the Amazonian poison dart frog; in this case failure to properly digest the casein protein produces a strong toxin with horrible effects on the child's developing nervous system.[1]

The upshot is that digesting, absorbing, and handling protein is a much trickier enterprise than the equivalent process for carbohydrate.

rejected by their recipient unless immunosuppressive drugs are given to ease their welcome. Even the relatively innocent reception you offer the foods you eat can be undermined by a reaction to the foreignness of the protein in a particular food, despite its subjection to the destructive processes of digestion. In other words, proteins are the basis of food allergy.

Thanks to nitrogen, proteins are so complex and varied that they provide no simple rule for recognition. Their one consistent feature is that they are richest in foods that come from animals. Even then, there are two important exceptions from the world of plants. One is a genus of blue-green algae called spirulina. This simple plant breaks the rules because it is nearly 70 percent protein. The other exception is beans, which are the seeds of the plant family known as legumes. (For a list of foods and a breakdown of their protein, carbohydrate, fat, calories, and other nutrients, see the charts at the end of this chapter.) Legumes, and particularly soybeans, have a special capacity to take nitrogen from the air and turn it into protein, thanks to an exceptional relationship with germs living on their roots that supply a necessary step in the transformation of atmospheric nitrogen into compounds the plants can utilize to form proteins.

Along with the higher protein content of soybeans goes a high overhead for getting them into edible condition. The trick to preparing soy is a method that allows it to be either fermented—meaning fed to germs before it's fed to you—or prepared in a way that makes it appetizing to the germs that live in your digestive tract so that you can properly break it down.

PROTEIN BURNS DIRTY

That the protein in your body originates in the nitrogen of the atmosphere also leads us to another important fact. Protein burns dirty. When carbohydrates are burned in your body they release carbon dioxide, energy, and water back to the forms from which they came. It's not so simple with nitrogen, which is one reason why a *strict* high protein diet is not good for you. And protein, unlike carbohydrate, is not a good source of fuel for your body's activities.

By burning dirty I mean that the nitrogen released in a protein fire is not returned to its original state but remains in a transitional and toxic form. The same is true in your body's metabolic fire; so consuming too much protein has different consequences from eating too much fat and carbohydrates, which will make you fat but not dirty.

This principle is easy to observe. When you singe your hair or your wool sweater, burn any animal product in a fire, or when animal products spoil or ferment, the results are particularly smelly. This contrasts with the fermentation of carbohydrates, like brewing beer, or the burning of wood, which burns clean.

Suppose you consume more nitrogen-containing substances, or proteins, during the day than your body needs to replace worn-out parts or, in the case of children, for growth. You do not just exhale nitrogen back into the air, as you do with the ingredients that went to make up carbohydrate. Nor do you store extra protein as fat. Instead, when you eat too much protein, your body goes through an elaborate process to get rid of the leftover nitrogen. The dirtiness of protein is a problem because getting rid of dirt—toxins, waste materials, or used-up molecules—is a metabolically expensive process in the body.

A high protein diet may be a good short-term bet for weight loss. But the *long term* costs of a high protein diet outweigh its benefits because of the cost of disposing of excess protein. By using the Circadian Diet to adjust the timing of your protein intake to optimize its use in the body at the appropriate times, you can achieve the same results. And you won't suffer the negative consequences of trying to burn protein for fuel.

WHY WE NEED PROTEIN

So if you're not eating protein to burn it as fuel, why do you need it? Obviously, if I'm asking you to eat most of your carbohydrates in the evening, then more fat and protein will automatically end up in your breakfast and lunch. But eating more of your protein during the day is not simply a default based on avoiding carbohydrates. Just as there are important reasons why your body needs carbohydrates at night, there are positive reasons for eating protein during the day. When I told Leslie to move most of her carbohydrates to the evening and eat protein in the morning and at lunch, good things happened to her. This was not just because she avoided morning carbohydrates—although that certainly had an impact—but because the protein itself had a clear effect. Protein supplies materials needed for one of the chief biochemical cycles of the daytime hours.

I gained my first appreciation of these cycles from the lectures of Dr. Charles Ehret when he explained the reasoning behind putting protein in the morning meal of the potentially jet lagged traveler. Protein provides a platform for the operation of the daytime chemistry of consciousness and action. Called adrenergic chemistry, this activity is named after the adrenal glands, which are a kind of branch office of the brain that lie atop (*ad*) the kidneys (*renal*). These glands are composed of an outer shell, or cortex, that produces, among other things, hydrocortisone, or cortisol. Every doctor knows that the cortisol level in the bloodstream changes significantly depending on the time of day; its peak is in the early morning hours, and its trough is in the evening. These levels are so time dependent that you cannot interpret a blood test for cortisol without knowing the time of day when the blood was taken.

Lying within the embrace of the cortex of each adrenal gland is the center core, or medulla, which produces an entirely different set of hormones. One of the principal products is known to most people by the term "adrenaline." Originally a trade name, adrenaline is now commonly used as another term for epinephrine, the hormone produced by this gland lying atop (*epi*) the kidney (*nephros*). Whether you use the Latin-rooted *adrenaline* or the Greek-rooted *epinephrine,* it's the same substance, essential for the state of consciousness and activity that humans must achieve during daylight hours.

The adrenergic phase is the biochemical process responsible for generating the substances that accompany cortisol and adrenaline at their highest levels into the bloodstream. Careful study of the amino acids employed in this chemistry and the enzymes that transform these amino acids into substances like epinephrine show that there is a morning window for this transaction within your body.[2] Dr. Ehret's prescription of protein in the morning was chosen on the basis of its presumed role as both a stimulus for opening the window and as a known provider of the substances needed once the window is open.

What it boils down to is that morning is the time for what you might call the "up" part of your body's chemistry. It's associated with the presence of higher levels of adrenaline, hydrocortisone, thyroid hormone, and other substances required for a state of alertness and activity. And because protein supplies the raw materials for adrenergic chemistry, failure to eat it in the morning leads to a general inefficiency in body chemistry, just like what would happen in an assembly line if the appropriate parts were not delivered at the right time and place. The results may be quite different in different people. But the common theme is not being sufficiently conscious, or "up," and it shows up in the level of mental alertness, attention span, concentration, and energy.

Notice the counterintuitive paradox here; everyone thinks that carbohydrates are for energy, so they find themselves puzzled when a breakfast of doughnuts and juice leaves them fuzzyheaded, exhausted, and hungry by midmorning. Taken in the evening, the same doughnuts and juice, however unhealthy, are appropriate and compatible with the nighttime activity of sleep.

Daytime levels of amino acids from protein are supposed to be higher than those at night. You cannot sustain healthy levels of amino acids during the day without daytime protein intake. Paradoxically, you need some of these amino acids for repair and growth at night, but it appears your body wants them delivered during the day shift. A particularly interesting twist is that tryptophan, an amino acid needed for sleep at night, is uniquely preserved in the bloodstream for nighttime use, demonstrating that your body has a mechanism for making materials delivered in the morning available at night, if they are needed.[3] Some people take tryptophan as a supplement with a carbohydrate snack at night to help them sleep. Many of them might be better off making sure they have a heavy protein load in the morning and letting their bodies take care of maintaining the supply of tryptophan for evening use.

For some time, scientists believed that day and night—or light and dark—were the only influences on the timing of human circadian chemistry. It is true that light and dark provide the strongest signals to keep your rhythm in synchrony with nature. But in the last twenty years it has been well established that all living creatures benefit from multiple timegivers whose power varies, depending on the individual and the circumstances. It's now clear that a combination of light, activity, and social stimulation, type and timing of food, and, in some creatures, heat and cold, profoundly affect the way an animal's body clock is set.[4] It's not clear precisely how consuming protein at breakfast and at noon benefited Leslie Hudson's chemistry. What is clear is that concentrating her protein intake early in the day helped her feel better.

When it comes to the timing of protein in the Circadian Diet, the basic principles pertain to sequencing and circadian cycles within your body; daytime biochemistry requires protein. As a result, you will feel better if you emphasize protein during the day and leave carbohydrates until evening. The experimental sciences and my patients' experiences provide support for this notion. And common sense dictates that we should do whatever we can to keep our chemistry operating efficiently, feeding ourselves the raw materials we need when our bodies need them.

CALORIC CONTENT AND COMPOSITION OF BREAKFAST FOODS

This list is sorted with the highest percent protein foods at the top. Each bar, which is sized proportionately for the number of calories per food, shows the percentage of total calories for protein, starch, sugar, fiber, unsaturated fat, and saturated fat. Labels on the left show the food, the number of calories per serving, and the serving size. The numbers appearing under the bars are grams per serving.

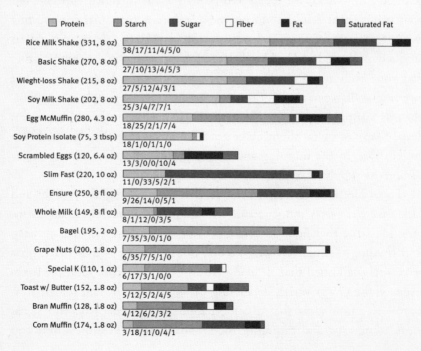

Protein   Starch   Sugar   Fiber   Fat   Saturated Fat

Rice Milk Shake (331, 8 oz) — 38/17/11/4/5/0
Basic Shake (270, 8 oz) — 27/10/13/4/5/3
Wieght-loss Shake (215, 8 oz) — 27/5/12/4/3/1
Soy Milk Shake (202, 8 oz) — 25/3/4/7/7/1
Egg McMuffin (280, 4.3 oz) — 18/25/2/1/7/4
Soy Protein Isolate (75, 3 tbsp) — 18/1/0/1/1/0
Scrambled Eggs (120, 6.4 oz) — 13/3/0/0/10/4
Slim Fast (220, 10 oz) — 11/0/33/5/2/1
Ensure (250, 8 fl oz) — 9/26/14/0/5/1
Whole Milk (149, 8 fl oz) — 8/1/12/0/3/5
Bagel (195, 2 oz) — 7/35/3/0/1/0
Grape Nuts (200, 1.8 oz) — 6/35/7/5/1/0
Special K (110, 1 oz) — 6/17/3/1/0/0
Toast w/ Butter (152, 1.8 oz) — 5/12/5/2/4/5
Bran Muffin (128, 1.8 oz) — 4/12/6/2/3/2
Corn Muffin (174, 1.8 oz) — 3/18/11/0/4/1

(cont'd)

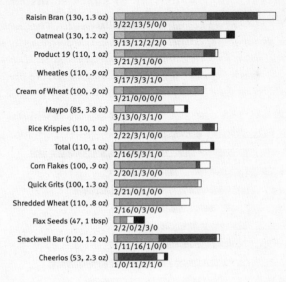

Raisin Bran (130, 1.3 oz) — 3/22/13/5/0/0
Oatmeal (130, 1.2 oz) — 3/13/12/2/2/0
Product 19 (110, 1 oz) — 3/21/3/1/0/0
Wheaties (110, .9 oz) — 3/17/3/3/1/0
Cream of Wheat (100, .9 oz) — 3/21/0/0/0/0
Maypo (85, 3.8 oz) — 3/13/0/3/1/0
Rice Krispies (110, 1 oz) — 2/22/3/1/0/0
Total (110, 1 oz) — 2/16/5/3/1/0
Corn Flakes (100, .9 oz) — 2/20/1/3/0/0
Quick Grits (100, 1.3 oz) — 2/21/0/1/0/0
Shredded Wheat (110, .8 oz) — 2/16/0/3/0/0
Flax Seeds (47, 1 tbsp) — 2/2/0/2/3/0
Snackwell Bar (120, 1.2 oz) — 1/11/16/1/0/0
Cheerios (53, 2.3 oz) — 1/0/11/2/1/0

CALORIC CONTENT AND COMPOSITION OF LUNCH FOODS

This list is sorted with the highest percent protein foods at the top. Each bar, which is sized proportionately for the number of calories per food, shows the percentage of total calories for protein, starch, sugar, fiber, unsaturated fat, and saturated fat. Labels on the left show the food, the number of calories per serving, and the serving size. The numbers appearing under the bars are grams per serving.

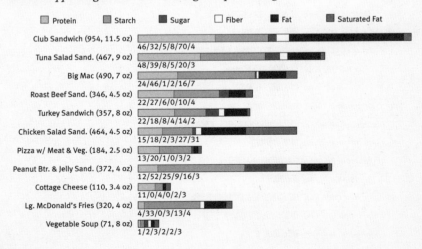

Legend: ▢ Protein ▢ Starch ▢ Sugar ▢ Fiber ▣ Fat ▢ Saturated Fat

Club Sandwich (954, 11.5 oz) — 46/32/5/8/70/4
Tuna Salad Sand. (467, 9 oz) — 48/39/8/5/20/3
Big Mac (490, 7 oz) — 24/46/1/2/16/7
Roast Beef Sand. (346, 4.5 oz) — 22/27/6/0/10/4
Turkey Sandwich (357, 8 oz) — 22/18/8/4/14/2
Chicken Salad Sand. (464, 4.5 oz) — 15/18/2/3/27/31
Pizza w/ Meat & Veg. (184, 2.5 oz) — 13/20/1/0/3/2
Peanut Btr. & Jelly Sand. (372, 4 oz) — 12/52/25/9/16/3
Cottage Cheese (110, 3.4 oz) — 11/0/4/0/2/3
Lg. McDonald's Fries (320, 4 oz) — 4/33/0/3/13/4
Vegetable Soup (71, 8 oz) — 1/2/3/2/2/3

CALORIC CONTENT AND COMPOSITION OF SNACK FOODS

This list is sorted with the highest percent protein foods at the top. Each bar, which is sized proportionately for the number of calories per food, shows the percentage of total calories for protein, starch, sugar, fiber, unsaturated fat, and saturated fat. Labels on the left show the food, the number of calories per serving, and the serving size. The numbers appearing under the bars are grams per serving.

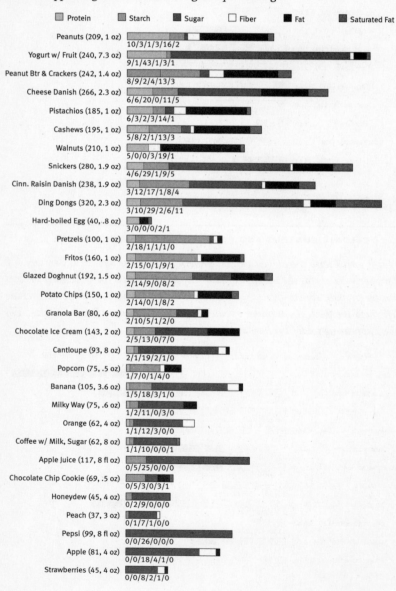

Protein   Starch   Sugar   Fiber   Fat   Saturated Fat

Peanuts (209, 1 oz)
10/3/1/3/16/2

Yogurt w/ Fruit (240, 7.3 oz)
9/1/43/1/3/1

Peanut Btr & Crackers (242, 1.4 oz)
8/9/2/4/13/3

Cheese Danish (266, 2.3 oz)
6/6/20/0/11/5

Pistachios (185, 1 oz)
6/3/2/3/14/1

Cashews (195, 1 oz)
5/8/2/1/13/3

Walnuts (210, 1 oz)
5/0/0/3/19/1

Snickers (280, 1.9 oz)
4/6/29/1/9/5

Cinn. Raisin Danish (238, 1.9 oz)
3/12/17/1/8/4

Ding Dongs (320, 2.3 oz)
3/10/29/2/6/11

Hard-boiled Egg (40, .8 oz)
3/0/0/0/2/1

Pretzels (100, 1 oz)
2/18/1/1/1/0

Fritos (160, 1 oz)
2/15/0/1/9/1

Glazed Doghnut (192, 1.5 oz)
2/14/9/0/8/2

Potato Chips (150, 1 oz)
2/14/0/1/8/2

Granola Bar (80, .6 oz)
2/10/5/1/2/0

Chocolate Ice Cream (143, 2 oz)
2/5/13/0/7/0

Cantloupe (93, 8 oz)
2/1/19/2/1/0

Popcorn (75, .5 oz)
1/7/0/1/4/0

Banana (105, 3.6 oz)
1/5/18/3/1/0

Milky Way (75, .6 oz)
1/2/11/0/3/0

Orange (62, 4 oz)
1/1/12/3/0/0

Coffee w/ Milk, Sugar (62, 8 oz)
1/1/10/0/0/1

Apple Juice (117, 8 fl oz)
0/5/25/0/0/0

Chocolate Chip Cookie (69, .5 oz)
0/5/3/0/3/1

Honeydew (45, 4 oz)
0/2/9/0/0/0

Peach (37, 3 oz)
0/1/7/1/0/0

Pepsi (99, 8 fl oz)
0/0/26/0/0/0

Apple (81, 4 oz)
0/0/18/4/1/0

Strawberries (45, 4 oz)
0/0/8/2/1/0

CALORIC CONTENT AND COMPOSITION OF DINNER FOODS

This list is sorted with the highest percent protein foods at the top. Each bar, which is sized proportionately for the number of calories per food, shows the percentage of total calories for protein, starch, sugar, fiber, unsaturated fat, and saturated fat. Labels on the left show the food, the number of calories per serving, and the serving size. The numbers appearing under the bars are grams per serving.

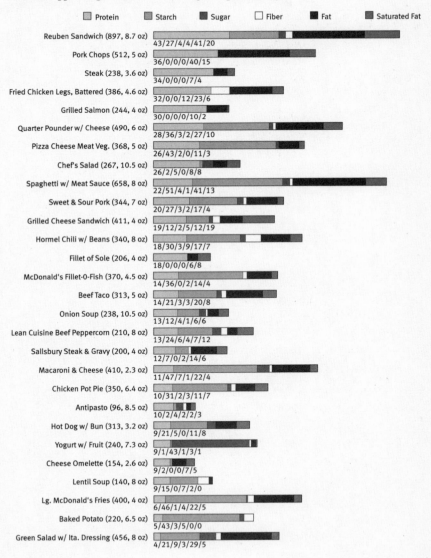

Legend: Protein | Starch | Sugar | Fiber | Fat | Saturated Fat

Reuben Sandwich (897, 8.7 oz) — 43/27/4/4/41/20
Pork Chops (512, 5 oz) — 36/0/0/0/40/15
Steak (238, 3.6 oz) — 34/0/0/0/7/4
Fried Chicken Legs, Battered (386, 4.6 oz) — 32/0/0/12/23/6
Grilled Salmon (244, 4 oz) — 30/0/0/0/10/2
Quarter Pounder w/ Cheese (490, 6 oz) — 28/36/3/2/27/10
Pizza Cheese Meat Veg. (368, 5 oz) — 26/43/2/0/11/3
Chef's Salad (267, 10.5 oz) — 26/2/5/0/8/8
Spaghetti w/ Meat Sauce (658, 8 oz) — 22/51/4/1/41/13
Sweet & Sour Pork (344, 7 oz) — 20/27/3/2/17/4
Grilled Cheese Sandwich (411, 4 oz) — 19/12/2/5/12/19
Hormel Chili w/ Beans (340, 8 oz) — 18/30/3/9/17/7
Fillet of Sole (206, 4 oz) — 18/0/0/0/6/8
McDonald's Fillet-O-Fish (370, 4.5 oz) — 14/36/0/2/14/4
Beef Taco (313, 5 oz) — 14/21/3/3/20/8
Onion Soup (238, 10.5 oz) — 13/12/4/1/6/6
Lean Cuisine Beef Peppercorn (210, 8 oz) — 13/24/6/4/7/12
Salisbury Steak & Gravy (200, 4 oz) — 12/7/0/2/14/6
Macaroni & Cheese (410, 2.3 oz) — 11/47/7/1/22/4
Chicken Pot Pie (350, 6.4 oz) — 10/31/2/3/11/7
Antipasto (96, 8.5 oz) — 10/2/4/2/2/3
Hot Dog w/ Bun (313, 3.2 oz) — 9/21/5/0/11/8
Yogurt w/ Fruit (240, 7.3 oz) — 9/1/43/1/3/1
Cheese Omelette (154, 2.6 oz) — 9/2/0/0/7/5
Lentil Soup (140, 8 oz) — 9/15/0/7/2/0
Lg. McDonald's Fries (400, 4 oz) — 6/46/1/4/22/5
Baked Potato (220, 6.5 oz) — 5/43/3/5/0/0
Green Salad w/ Ita. Dressing (456, 8 oz) — 4/21/9/3/29/5

(cont'd)

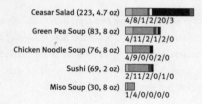

Ceasar Salad (223, 4.7 oz)
4/8/1/2/20/3

Green Pea Soup (83, 8 oz)
4/11/2/1/2/0

Chicken Noodle Soup (76, 8 oz)
4/9/0/0/2/0

Sushi (69, 2 oz)
2/11/2/0/1/0

Miso Soup (30, 8 oz)
1/4/0/0/0/0

24:00
25:00
01:00
02:00
03:00
04:00
05:00
06:00
07:00
08:00
09:00
10:00
11:00
12:00
13:00
14:00
15:00
16:00
17:00
18:00
19:00
20:00
21:00
22:00
23:00
24:00
25:00
01:00

CHAPTER

6

The Rhythmic Shake and the Ten Rules of the Circadian Diet

t's been my experience that it is probably easier to get people to change their religion than to alter their diet. After all, in our own society we see people many generations removed from their native lands still eating the food typical of their culture, despite having changed many of their other cultural habits, including the very language they speak.

The Circadian Diet alters *when* you eat certain foods rather than *what* you eat, assuming you eat a reasonably healthy diet. You'll find that you can make the diet work even if you've been discouraged by the rigid rules and complex calculations you may have had to do with other diet programs.

To get a jumpstart, I recommend the Rhythmic Shake, which I consider the keystone of the diet. The simplicity and efficiency of the shake especially appeal to me as a physician because for many people it brings immediate results. This drink is something you can have for breakfast—and, if you prefer, for lunch. For most people, the shake provides a simple way to achieve the dietary changes that I prescribe without learning a whole new way to cook, shop, or eat.

The shake is high in protein, so it reinforces a healthy circadian rhythm that in turn bolsters other rhythms—brain waves, cardiovascular tempo, breathing, and the menstrual cycle—in your body. Since it includes soy protein and flaxseed fiber, the shake provides the information your body needs to beneficially modulate your hormone chemistry. If you make it with yogurt, it also encourages a normal population of germs in your digestive tract. Unlike other foods that are "good for you," the shake is tasty. And it can be a vehicle for adding other healthy phytonutrients to your daily diet.

I know that changing what you eat for breakfast is not an easy thing to do. I myself have never been a "shake" kind of person. But now that I understand and have experienced the benefits, both personally and through my patients, I am committed to the Rhythmic Shake. Despite having to change their eating habits, most of my patients have adapted readily to the shake because they experience such an immediate, dramatic improvement of daytime energy, mood, and clear-headedness when they try it, *and* since they understand what they'll gain in terms of reduced cancer and other health risks.

The recipe for the Basic Shake follows. I also offer variations you can use to suit your tastes or allergic sensitivities, to lose weight, or to tackle insulin resistance. Feel free to experiment with other fruits or flavorings, like vanilla. In the summer, try adding ice to the blender for a cooler, crunchier alternative. And if you prefer a warm breakfast during cold winter weather, put the shake in a saucepan and heat it on the stove. It will thicken to form a tasty, warming, puddinglike dish similar to oatmeal. And warming it just to the point to make it nice to eat on a cold morning is not enough to damage the flaxseed oil.

THE BASIC SHAKE

If you're a reasonably healthy person who simply wants to have more energy during the day and avoid drowsiness in the late morning and afternoon, the Basic Shake is for you. If you don't need to control your weight or want to gain weight, you can add the shake to a breakfast that contains other sources of protein such as fish, meat, eggs, or cheese. Alternatively, you can make and drink more of the shake.

If you're used to eating a quick breakfast of juice, toast, bagels or other bread with jam, and tea or coffee, it's probable that no book is going to motivate you to start eating eggs, meat, and fish in the morning. Given what's at stake in terms of both the immediate rewards and the reduced risks of disease, maybe you're willing to add the shake to your high carbohydrate breakfast. I'm not going to lie to you; you're overloading the carbohydrates. The addition of the shake will not raise the percentage of the protein content of your breakfast as much as I would recommend, but it will certainly be better than doing nothing. You may experience some of the benefits of getting the protein load in the morning, especially when it comes to avoiding that wiped-out feeling during the late morning or in the afternoon. And consuming soy and flaxseed daily will provide you with protection against reproductive cancers. But to get the full benefits of the Circadian Diet, you'll have to go farther and limit the carbohydrates you're consuming.

If you have a tendency to gain weight, you can make the Basic Shake your whole breakfast. You'll feel satisfied, and at the same time you'll avoid the late morning letdown that often occurs when you eat a lot of carbohydrates at breakfast. To gradually shed some pounds, you can try the Weight Loss Shake or the Soy Milk Shake. (See chapter 11 for more about weight loss.)

The main ingredients of the Rhythmic Shake are milk, yogurt, ground flaxseeds, soy protein isolate, and fruit. I use milk and yogurt for the Basic Shake because milk is an excellent source of protein and calcium, as well as a convenient and preferred beverage for many, and yogurt contains lactobacillus (acidophilus), which helps maintain or restore the healthy flora, or germ population, of your intestines. (This is only true of yogurt that contains a live culture.) Blueberries are low in calories and rich in taste and provide valuable nutrients.

The flaxseed powder provides a little extra texture and acts as a thickener, which explains why the shake will become almost too thick to drink if you don't consume it right away. In terms of quantity, the oil in the flaxseeds is a minor ingredient; nor is it as closely connected as protein to the day and night cycle. But its contribution to the shake is not trivial; that little bit of oil may be enough to restore luster to your skin, manageability to your hair, and flexibility to your cell membranes and to reduce your risk for a variety of malignant inflammatory diseases. (See chapter 7 for more about fats and oils.) You can buy whole flaxseeds at the health food store; store them in a covered container in the refrigerator. Grind them in a coffee or spice grinder. You can keep the freshly ground flaxseed powder in the grinder for a day or two at most; longer than that and they may become rancid.

For protein, I recommend soy protein isolate, a relatively bland-tasting, tan-colored powder that is the most concentrated protein product derived from soy. No other soy protein product, including soy protein concentrate, provides as much protein. You can buy soy protein isolate at the health-food store.

If you are sensitive to soy, you'll want to substitute another vegetable protein, such as rice protein (see the recipe for the Rice Milk Shake).

The Basic Shake
(270 Calories)

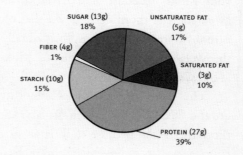

3 ounces whole milk

3 ounces regular yogurt

1 tablespoon ground flaxseeds

3 tablespoons soy protein isolate

¼ cup blueberries, fresh or frozen

Put the yogurt and milk in a blender. With the blender on low speed, add ground flaxseeds, soy protein isolate, and blueberries. Increase the speed until ingredients are well blended.

The Weight Loss Shake
(215 Calories)

If you are trying to limit calories, substitute skim milk and low fat or non-fat yogurt. You can see from the pie chart that the Weight Loss Shake using low fat yogurt provides 55 fewer calories than the Basic Shake. When you're trying to lose weight, every calorie counts, so feel free to use nonfat yogurt if you prefer. (Check out the Soy Milk Shake if you want even fewer calories.) You can also reduce calories by making a smaller amount of shake, but be sure to use the *full amount* of soy protein powder and flaxseed. A little bit of fruit will go a long way toward improving the taste of the Weight Loss Shake without adding substantially to the calories.

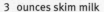

3 ounces skim milk

3 ounces light (low fat or no fat) yogurt

1 tablespoon ground flaxseeds

3 tablespoons soy protein isolate

¼ cup blueberries, fresh or frozen

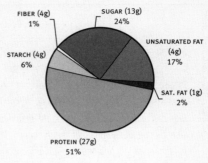

Follow directions for the Basic Shake.

Notice that the sugar content of the weight loss shake (13 grams) is about the same as the rice milk shake (11 grams). However, sugar as a percentage of total calories in the weight loss shake is more (24 percent compared to 14 percent) because the total calories in the weight loss shake are fewer.

The Soy Milk Shake
(202 Calories)

If you're sensitive to milk and milk products, you'll have to substitute another beverage for the milk and yogurt in the shake. Soy milk, the watery solution obtained by mashing up soybeans in water and straining off the liquid, is the first choice. If you are sensitive to cow's milk but not lactose intolerant, you may be able to use goat's milk.

This is the lowest calorie shake, so you can also use it to lose weight.

6 ounces soy milk

1 tablespoon ground flaxseeds

3 tablespoons soy protein isolate

¼ cup blueberries, fresh or frozen

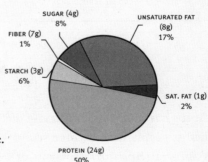

Follow directions for the Basic Shake.

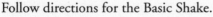

SENSITIVITY TO MILK

Milk sensitivity comes in three forms. Many people are lactose intolerant, or sensitive to lactose to one degree or another. Lactose is the sweet ingredient found in the milk of all mammals. People who are lactose intolerant lack the enzyme that splits lactose into its two components, galactose and glucose, during digestion. This process has to occur in order for lactose to enter the bloodstream for use by the body. If it doesn't happen, the lactose is not only useless but actually mischievous, because there are germs normally found in the lower part of the digestive system that like to eat it. When they do, they produce gas and cause cramps and other changes that may evoke a watery diarrhea.

If you can't overcome the effects by consuming milk that has been treated with Lactaid®, which predigests the lactose, then milk and milk products should be avoided.

Distinct from lactose intolerance is a second problem: milk allergy. An allergy is a bad reaction to a small amount of a substance that doesn't bother most other people. While a lactose intolerance produces mostly intestinal complaints, milk allergy can produce just about any symptom—everything from depression to hyperactivity, from diarrhea to eczema, and from wheezing to sneezing. Some reactions to milk can be tested and confirmed by doctors; others are more mysterious. But milk sensitivity is high on the list of possibilities I consider when a patient has a mysterious symptom of any kind.

The third possible problem with milk is sensitivity to casein, one of the main proteins in milk. Casein sensitivity may involve an immune system reaction to the milk protein. On the other hand, sometimes casein causes trouble because of the peptides that arise during its digestion and provide troublesome false messages to your body.

The Rice Milk Shake
(331 Calories)

As soy has entered the American diet in the last couple of decades, a number of people have become sensitive to it, reacting with gastrointestinal, skin, and respiratory problems or other expressions of allergy. If you are sensitive to animal milk and to soy, you can substitute rice milk and another vegetable protein: rice. When rice is milled, the chaff or outer coating of the whole rice grain is removed, leaving behind the kernel that we consume as white rice. The small amount of protein that makes up any cereal grain lies within the outer coating and can be concentrated from the chaff into a powder that is essentially pure protein, even though it was derived from a source that was mostly carbohydrate. You can buy rice protein at the health food store.

If you want to replace other substances that you will be missing by eliminating the soy, your best bet is to increase the flaxseed powder, because flaxseed contains the same types of beneficial phytonutrients present in soy. On the other hand, if you keep increasing the flaxseed content of your shake, it will get so thick that it's quite hard to consume except with a spoon. It does, once placed in the freezer, make good popsicles that appeal to children (see chapter 13 for popsicle recipe). In any case, don't exceed 3 tablespoons of flaxseed powder per day; larger amounts can cause thyroid problems.

6 ounces rice milk

1 tablespoon ground flaxseeds

3 tablespoons rice protein

¼ cup blueberries, fresh or frozen

Follow directions for the Basic Shake.

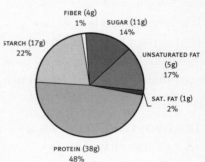

USING THE SHAKE TO REGULATE INSULIN LEVELS

If you scored over 20 on the Insulin Resistance Checklist in chapter 4, or if you've been told by your doctor that you have hyperinsulinemia, insulin resistance, or Syndrome X, the Circadian Prescription is for you. Your insulin levels will come down if you limit how frequently you eat carbohydrates. This means restricting most of your carbohydrates to the evening.

When your breakfast shake is as low as possible in carbohydrates, your insulin levels will fall, relieving you of the symptoms as well as the risk factors associated with insulin resistance. You should gradually substitute the high protein shake for the high carbohydrate breakfast you're probably used to eating. The key word here is "gradually." You can't do this all of a sudden. If you plunged into the program tomorrow by eating a high protein shake and very few carbohydrates for breakfast, your elevated insulin levels would cause intolerable carbohydrate cravings in the morning. When people switch to a high protein regimen, cold turkey, it usually takes about three to four weeks for carbohydrate cravings to subside.

Instead, take a number of weeks to gradually reduce the amount of carbohydrate in your shake. Follow the Basic Shake recipe for two weeks and then switch to the Weight Loss Shake. Stay on that for another two weeks. When you're comfortable, move on to the Soy Milk Shake, which is the variation with the lowest carbohydrate content.

The idea is to find a point where the taste of the shake is still acceptable, so you're not getting up every morning to face something that you find unpalatable. On the other hand, remember that your goal involves much higher and more immediate stakes than for most people. Your aim is to reverse a highly malignant process involving uncontrolled insulin levels that has a major impact on your immediate and long-term health.

If you are planning to eat more for breakfast or lunch than the shake, your choices should be limited to high fiber vegetables and lean meats.

THE BOOSTER SHAKE: ADDING MORE PHYTONUTRIENTS TO THE RHYTHMIC SHAKE

By now you know that phytonutrients are an important subplot of the Circadian Prescription story. I've included soy protein and flaxseed fiber in the shake for their many benefits, but especially because the phytonutrients they contain improve reproductive health and lower the risk of breast, prostate, and other related cancers.

Phytonutrients, however, are not limited to flaxseed and rye fiber, or soybeans. On the contrary, in the last several years scientific knowledge about the beneficial effects of the phytonutrients in many foods has exploded, demonstrating along the way that these substances are much more concentrated in certain plants than in others.

The best bet is to eat a varied diet. However, we Americans tend to eat a very limited number of foods. And many of the foods we eat have been extracted from their plant source, rather than consumed as part of the plant itself, leaving behind most of the nutritionally important proteins, carbohydrates, vitamins, minerals, and phytonutrients.

If you're not about to increase the variety of foods you eat, the Rhythmic Shake, no matter what variation you use, can serve as a convenient vehicle for adding plant-derived phytonutrients to your diet. The difficulty is deciding which ones to choose.

The scientific literature on phytonutrients contains a surprisingly long list of things that seem to be good for you. A short list of substances that have recently received scientific attention includes: green tea; gingko; wheat grass, barley grass, alfalfa sprouts, and oats; licorice root; ginseng; spirulina and chlorella; various other algaes and seaweeds; astragalus; echinacea; ginger; soy lecithin; acerola berry; beet juice; spinach; octacosonols: royal jelly or bee pollen; vitamin E; pectins; milk thistle; grape pips; and bilberry. If you were to invest in a bottle of each and line them up next to your blender, you'd go crazy every time you tried to make a shake.

Instead, I recommend using one of several brands of green food concentrates that contain many of the substances I just mentioned; you can find them in your health food store. Popular brands are: Progreens (Allergy Research), Gary Null's Green Stuff, Green Magma (Green Foods Corporation), Greens and More (Solgar), Kyogreens (Wakunaga) By adding a scoop of such a concentrate to your shake you can cover some of the nutritional bases that have been discovered over the last few years.

BEYOND THE RHYTHMIC SHAKE: THE TEN RULES OF THE CIRCADIAN DIET

The Rhythmic Shake is a first step that incorporates many of the diet's basic principles; it gives you a fast, easy way to get going on the diet. The rules of the diet are also quite simple. They require neither great inconvenience for you nor drastic changes in what you eat. And the Circadian Diet is flexible; it's more important to understand the basic framework than a whole lot of details.

RULE 1: Put protein in your morning meal, snacks, and lunch. Emphasize fish, eggs, milk products (for those who can handle them), nuts, peanuts, soy, poultry, beans, and meat.

If you don't eat breakfast, there's something wrong. Morning hunger is a natural and healthy reflection of the proper functioning of your body's chemistry. Remarkably, your body is capable of sustaining your blood sugar at higher levels during the night than during the day, but as soon as you awaken and become active your metabolic need for food changes dramatically and should give you a reliable signal to eat.

If you are not hungry in the morning, you may be caught in a vicious cycle in which your rhythms are out of whack and that very wackiness is depriving you of hunger. Beginning to take protein in the morning may help set things straight, even if the quantities involved are small. It's fine to be gentle with your body. Remember, my recommendations are meant to provide gradual, healthy, and permanent changes.

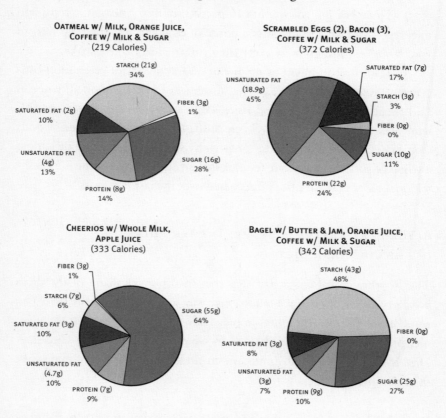

Nutritional breakdown of four breakfast choices. The traditional scrambled eggs, bacon, and coffee breakfast, minus the toast, gives the best bargain in terms of high protein and low carbohydrate. The other choices are mostly sugar and starch. Note that "sugar" includes natural sugars that are part of milk (lactose) or apple juice (sucrose and fructose), as well as added sweeteners.

The Rhythmic Shake is the easiest way to get protein into your morning meal, and it brings the benefits of its phytonutrient-rich ingredients. However, other protein-rich foods will provide results similar to the shake in terms of daytime alertness and energy. The only food whose density of protein is equivalent to soy protein (or the rice protein substitute) is egg white, which is essentially 100 percent protein. The protein content of most other protein rich-foods ranges between 25 and 85 percent.

Researchers consider a high protein diet to be in the range of 40 to 60 percent protein,[1] so please don't get the idea that your breakfast or lunch should consist of 100 percent protein. I am suggesting, however, that your body's chemistry and rhythms will give you a much smoother ride if you approach this range.

RULE 2: Move most of your carbohydrates from breakfast, lunch, and morning snacks to the evening.

After 4:00 p.m., your goal is to cut back on protein and emphasize healthy carbohydrate-rich foods like pasta, bread, potato, sweet potato and other starchy vegetables, whole cereal grains, seeds, sprouts and fruit. You can even include a moderate amount of sweets.

It's not possible or desirable to transfer all the carbohydrates that you eat from morning to evening; instead, I'm talking about emphasis. If you are eating a breakfast based on rolls, coffee, and juice and a high carbohydrate lunch, you will feel better simply by adding protein in the morning and at noon. However, this may also substantially increase the calories you are eating at those meals, which is not desirable unless you are trying to gain weight. You can avoid this problem and experience more dramatic results if you save most of your rolls, juice, fruit, and other carbohydrates for dinner. By the same token, if you're already eating a lot of carbohydrates in the evening, don't feel any obligation to eat your breakfast juice and rolls as well as your pasta and dessert; research has shown that weight gain is promoted more easily by food consumption late in the day than early in the day.

Nor do you have to completely cut protein out of your evening meal. Scientists have not completely resolved the question of how daytime protein intake is reserved for nighttime cell multiplication, growth, and repair. It appears that the morning intake of protein is set aside or put in

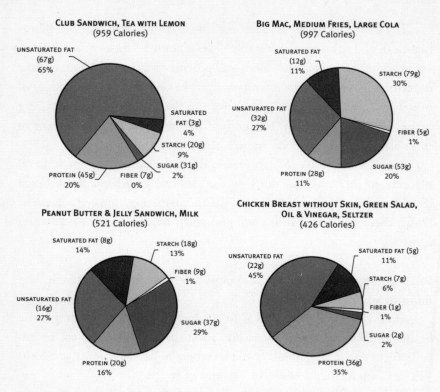

Nutritional breakdown of four meal choices. The only really high protein (35 percent), low carbohydrate (8 percent starch and sugar) choice is the chicken breast, which also has about one-half the calories of the club sandwich or Big Mac. Furthermore, even though the Big Mac and peanut butter sandwich are each based on a relatively high protein ingredient, they are both essentially high carbohydrate meals.

line for nighttime use. In contrast, when it comes to carbohydrates, Alain Reinberg, a foremost circadian researcher, points out that "one can expect that food as fuel might to some extent be 'wasted' when taken in the morning and 'stored' when taken in the evening."[2] The basis for Dr. Reinberg's statement is that carbohydrate taken in the morning dissipates during the day; when taken in the evening it is sustained for nighttime use.

RULE 3: Eat plenty of fresh vegetables to take advantage of their fiber, antioxidants, and phytochemicals, which have been shown to provide protection against a growing number of diseases, including high blood pressure, heart disease, cancer, and macular degeneration.[3]

TIMING YOUR VEGETABLES

Circadian neutral vegetables

Leaves are fibrous and not starchy, so green leafy vegetables (for example, lettuce, spinach, watercress, beet greens, chard) can be eaten any time of day; the same is true for stems, like celery, and flowers, such as artichokes and asparagus.

Cruciferous vegetables, such as cabbage, bok choy, broccoli, collards, kale, Brussels sprouts, and cauliflower, contain ample fiber and abundant phytonutrients. The body of scientific evidence supporting their health benefits is enormous.[4]

Vegetables with seeds in pods are high in fiber, even though the seeds themselves contain a fair amount of starch. Most such seeds are in the legume family (beans) and are therefore good sources of protein, which compensates for their being rich in carbohydrates and fat. You can treat nuts the same as you do legumes; in fact, nuts make excellent daytime snacks.

In botanical terms, pumpkins, squash, cucumbers, tomatoes, peppers, and eggplants are fruits, though we treat them like vegetables. Most of their weight is water, not starch, and what's left is mostly fiber; you can eat them at any meal.

Bulbs, like onions, garlic, leeks, and other members of the Allium family, are also fibrous and can be eaten any time.

Sweet corn is a seed that people mistake for a vegetable. It really belongs with the cereal grains, which are starchy and should be eaten later in the day.

Starchy Vegetables

For the most part, try to eat vegetables from tubers and roots in the evening. The true root vegetables—carrots, beets, rutabagas, turnips, parsnips, and radishes—are not as starchy as the tubers, so you can eat them in small amounts during the day. But tubers, such as potatoes, cassava (tapioca, manioc, yucca), sweet potatoes, and yams are almost pure starch and should be restricted to evening.

The right time of day to eat a particular vegetable depends on how much of its contents is fiber and how much is starch. Most vegetables are fibrous, so they are circadian neutral—you can eat them at any meal. Starchy vegetables should be reserved for evening. How can you tell which is which? A good rule of thumb is to look at what part of the plant the vegetable comes from. See the box for guidelines.

RULE 4: Eat plenty of fresh fruit, but save most of it for evening.

Like vegetables, fruits are rich in vitamins, minerals, and other nutrients that help prevent disease. But they also contain large amounts of natural sugars.

Raw fruit is sweet enough to raise your blood sugar and stimulate insulin production, but it has enough fiber content to blunt those effects. Therefore, I won't discourage you from eating an apple with your lunch or putting some blueberries in your shake. Still, fruits, and particularly sauces and juices prepared from them, can cause mischief with respect to your carbohydrate chemistry, and it's more likely to happen when you consume them early in the day. If you can, postpone fruit until late afternoon or evening.

RULE 5: Avoid caffeine except at around 4:00 p.m., when it is circadian neutral.

Caffeine, and similar compounds found in coffee, tea, or chocolate, has as strong an influence on circadian rhythms as any over-the-counter drug yet discovered. The reason for not drinking coffee or tea in the morning is that it tends to shift your circadian clock in the direction of lengthening your day. When you drink caffeine in the evening, it tends to shift your clock in the direction of shortening your day. Caffeine may help you adjust to jet lag, but it is otherwise a disconcerting influence if you want to strengthen your circadian rhythms or if your rhythms are disturbed. If you're going to drink coffee or tea, the only time of day when it is circadian neutral is British tea time, around 4:00 p.m.[5]

The circadian effects of caffeine are independent of its well-known stimulant effect. Drinking coffee in the morning may affect your sleep at night, even though the caffeine in your system has long gone, because it has thrown off your body clock, which governs the quality of your sleep. On the other hand, people who are very sensitive to the stimulant effects of caffeine may find that even the circadian neutral time of 4:00 p.m. is too late in the day to avoid disturbing their sleep.

RULE 6: Limit consumption of alcohol to the evening.

All forms of alcohol—wine, beer, and liquor—are highly concentrated carbohydrates. If you drink alcohol, do it in the evening. However, consuming large amounts of alcohol—to the point of intoxication—will cause a total disruption in your circadian rhythm, no matter when you drink it.[6]

RULE 7: Eliminate artificial sweeteners and diet drinks.

You're probably aware that the informational roller coaster on artificial sweeteners has had particularly sharp ups and downs. The role of saccharine, cyclamates, and aspartame as potential miracles or poisons receives periodic attention in the scientific literature and the popular press. Some of the world's top neuroscientists, such as Richard Wurtman and his colleague John Fernstrom at the Massachusetts Institute of Technology, have pointed to aspartame's potential interference with neurotransmitter function,[7] and indeed the vigilant practitioner will occasionally find patients whose symptoms are relieved by abstinence from aspartame.

I have been surprised to find patients who seemed to suffer the same adverse effects from any artificial sweetener—going back to the days when cyclamates were available. How could it be that such different substances produce similar symptoms in a given person? I've also wondered whether there's anything in artificial sweeteners that might cause mischief for all of us.

Whether something causes cancer or interferes with neurotransmitters is certainly not irrelevant, but the main issue with artificial sweeteners is trickery. In the natural world, sweet taste is exclusively connected to edible substances. A molecular spot on your taste buds actually measures the distance, unique to sugars, between certain atoms. This permits your tongue to report the arrival of safe and edible sugars to your brain with absolute reliability. Absolute, that is, until scientists devised molecules, at first by chance (saccharine) and later by design (aspartame), whose atomic distances exactly mimic those of their truly sweet counterparts, the sugars.

Your first sip of a diet soda tells your brain, which has never had any reason to doubt the tongue's truthfulness in this regard, "here comes sugar." Given sugar's importance as the ultimate currency in your food economy, your tongue's treacherous lie raises metabolic expectations and mobilizes vital processes. It's as if you made a date for dinner, told your date to order for you, and then failed to show up. Your brain tells your body to get insulin because sugar is on its way. Insulin levels begin to rise, but what you've imbibed is empty of the very calories the insulin is there to distribute. The insulin grabs whatever real sugar is available and pushes it into your cells. This causes your blood sugar to drop, providing a truthful signal to your brain that you need sugar. This cycle is the real roller coaster in the artificial sweetener story. And it is the mechanism behind the diet soda habit that I see in so many people who tease their metabolism while quenching their thirst.

RULE 8: Consume healthy oils.

Fat is generally circadian neutral, but some fats are healthier than others. For cooking, no other oil can compete with olive oil in terms of its high levels of desirable monounsaturated fats and its low levels of saturated fat, although canola and walnut oil are also healthy choices.

Because they provide such significant health benefits, the intake of some oils is virtually medicinal. These include fish oil concentrates containing the longer chain omega-3 fatty acids and flaxseed oil, which is the richest source for the fatty acid that is the mother of the omega-3 family. (See chapter 7 for more about fats and oils.) Including fish in your diet is a good way to increase your consumption of these essential omega-3 oils. If you like, you can experiment with flaxseed oil in salad dressing or in other culinary uses where it is not subjected to high heat. I have to warn you, though, that I don't find it a particularly palatable addition to foods.

You may benefit from fish oil or flaxseed oil supplements. If so, remember that bile, which is important for digesting fat, flows from your liver into your gallbladder during sleep, so first thing in the morning is when your gallbladder is best able to handle an intake of fat or oils. Therefore, if you're taking supplements of flaxseed oil or fish oil, breakfast time is the best time to take them.

RULE 9: Drink eight glasses of water a day.

Most people spend much more time thinking about eating than about drinking. But getting enough fluids is essential to your health. Water is the basis for all bodily fluids. Every cell and organ function depends on it; it is also necessary to keep food moving through the digestive tract and for proper elimination. You do get some fluid from the foods you eat, but most researchers agree that adults require eight glasses a day to replace what is lost in normal body functions. Anything that increases fluid loss, like exercise or illness—especially fever, diarrhea, vomiting, infections, and burns—also increases your need for water. Unlike juice, soda, and sports drinks, water contains no carbohydrates. It is also rapidly absorbed by the body.

RULE 10: Eat regularly.

Staying in harmony with Nature is not always easy. Remember that your internal body clock is quite stubbornly set at about twenty-four hours, and every day you depend on timegivers to keep you in synchrony with your environment. Exposure to light was the first timegiver recognized as a synchronizer; all things being equal, it might be the strongest. All things, however, are not equal. We are all caught in a stream of influences that may compete with light, and with each other, to reset our clocks forward or backward depending on the intensity and time of day of exposure. Many of us living in northern latitudes and working indoors receive little exposure to direct outdoor sunlight. Moreover, exposure to artificial light may act as a significant desynchronizing influence.[8] The relative decrease in the dose and, therefore, the power of light only increases the importance of food as a synchronizer. Regular eating helps keep your body functioning on time, and your chemistry will appreciate the regularly scheduled delivery of the materials it needs. The best schedule for eating is breakfast at 7:00 a.m., lunch at midday, and supper in the early evening. You can vary these times, but the key is to be faithful to your routine.

Now that you have the recipes for the Rhythmic Shake and the rules for the diet, you have the essential components of the Circadian Prescription. In the chapters ahead I'll outline the other factors that come into play in achieving rhythmic integration and optimum health.

24:00
25:00
01:00
02:00
03:00
04:00
05:00
06:00
07:00
08:00
09:00
10:00
11:00
12:00
13:00
14:00
15:00
16:00
17:00
18:00
19:00
20:00
21:00
22:00
23:00
24:00
25:00
01:00

CHAPTER

7

Miracle Fats

F ats are considered neutral when it comes to circadian rhythm, but they are so important to your health that it would be remiss for me to leave them out. Along with protein and carbohydrates, fat is one of the three basic components of food. But the beneficial and negative aspects of fat have been the subject of much debate and confusion.

We've been told for the last twenty years how harmful fat is. The real issue, however, is not the total fat in your diet but which fats you eat. There are good fats and bad fats. In fact, by avoiding fat in general you're in danger of depriving yourself of critical nutrients and substantially increasing your risk factors for a variety of illnesses.

I'll start by clearing up the terminology that confuses so many people. "Lipids" is a technical term applied to all fatty molecules that are distinguished by their insolubility in water. The word "oil" simply designates a fat that tends to be liquid or runny at room temperature. Oil that comes out of the ground as petroleum (*petro* is rock; *oleo* is oil), and all the products that come from it, were originally vegetable oil, formed by living plants whose decay over millions of years deposited oily residues that stayed in one place because oil doesn't mix with water.

A fatty acid is the smallest unit of fat; it does not have a sour taste like vinegar or lemon juice, so it is only acid in a technical chemical sense. A molecule that consists of three fatty acids attached by another small molecule like three big prongs on a small fork, is called a triglyceride, and this is what constitutes your body's fat stores; in other words, it's what we're talking about when we say someone is fat. Another important location of your body fat is in the membranes in and around every cell in your body. This fat is in the form of diglycerides (two fatty acids held together by the same small molecule that holds together triglycerides).

Cholesterol is not a fatty acid but a complex molecule used by animals as a component of cell membranes and as raw material for making steroid hormones (e.g., cortisol, testosterone, estrogen, and progesterone). Thus, all animal fat and tissue contains cholesterol. Cholesterol appears in your body as a result of eating it or because you synthesize it as a necessary part of your own healthy chemistry. Because cholesterol forms part of the harmful deposits of vascular disease, it has been blamed for those diseases. But I believe that within the next few years it will be found that cholesterol is a participant, not the real culprit.

The term "fatty acid" is more scientifically specific than just saying "oil"; practically speaking, oil, fat, grease, lard, butter, margarine, and shortening are the foods that bring fatty acids into your body. But for our purposes, the differences among fats, oils, and fatty acids are negligible.

OMEGA-3 AND OMEGA-6 FATTY ACIDS

There are a variety of fatty acids in foods, including two families, the omega-3 family and the omega-6 family, that are called essential because your body cannot make them without the raw materials in food. These two types of fatty acids are in turn the sole raw materials for making a whole set of your body's key hormones (prostaglandins). These two essential fatty acids are also the main contributors of flexibility to your cell membranes.

Omega-3 and omega-6 fatty acids have a tiny but crucial structural difference—the position of a double bond either three or six positions in from the omega end of the molecule—which accounts for their names.

The best sources of good fatty acids are the polyunsaturated omega-3 oils found in flaxseed, fish, and walnut oils, as well as canola oil, which is made from a special breed of rapeseed developed to be rich in omega-3 fatty acids. The monounsaturated oils found in olive oil also contain good fatty acids.

The dietary source that provides all the omega-3 family of fatty acids is alpha-linolenic acid (ALA). Over the last few decades, our diets have become increasingly deficient in ALA. Without special supplements of ALA or other members of the omega-3 family, like fish oils, deficiencies of omega-3 fatty acids may occur, causing stiffening, cracking, flaking, and dryness of your hair, nails, and skin. A sampling of recent studies shows that omega-3 oils also provide protection against a number of serious conditions:[1]

- The types of cardiovascular disease people associate with high cholesterol are prevented by a diet that is high in omega-3 oils.

- Patients suffering from rheumatoid arthritis get a statistically significant benefit from taking supplements of these oils as compared with those who received a placebo.

- A study of breast cancer in mice showed essentially 100 percent protection in cancer-prone mice supplemented with flaxseed or fish oils, as compared to a rapid death rate in controls and in mice fed other oils; human studies have demonstrated the relevance of these data to women.

- Omega-3 oils have been shown to help asthma, attention deficit disorder, diabetes, depression, insulin resistance, menstrual cramps, stroke, hypertension, multiple sclerosis, psoriasis, and eczema.

I first learned about the far-reaching effects of omega-3 oils twenty years ago, when I saw Melissa Black. This nine-year-old girl had been seeing a family therapist with her parents for three years. The psychiatrist could not find anything about her care or development that could explain her mood changes and uncontrollable outbursts of rage. During the same three years she had also been consulting a dermatologist because her feet were plagued by painful recurrent cracks, fissures, and a tendency for the skin to come off in sheets. The constant application of various skin conditioners and steroids remedied neither these symptoms nor the shiny, delicate appearance of the skin on her feet. Every night she went through a ritual of slathering steroid cream on her feet and covering them with white cotton socks.

At the beginning of Melissa's treatments, the dry, flaking and cracking condition of her feet was a clue that a fatty acid problem might be causing symptoms in her feet that were not evident in other parts of her skin and hair and that this problem might also be affecting the functioning of her central nervous system. From lab tests, I found that she was extremely low in alpha-linolenic acid. I prescribed a daily supplement of a tablespoon of flaxseed oil, which has a rich concentration of ALA. Within a few weeks her skin cleared up and her tantrums disappeared.

FATS MAKE CELL MEMBRANES

How can one treatment cure both itchy scaly feet and tantrums? To understand how fats affect so many different aspects of health, you need to see how they work at a cellular level. Your body is made up of a hundred trillion tiny packages of life called cells. Each cell is like an egg in which the yolk is the nucleus and the white is the cytoplasm. There is no shell; instead, the outer covering of the "egg" is an ultrathin membrane composed of two layers of oil molecules.

Inside this egglike structure, rather than the clear jelly you find inside a hen's egg, is a complicated arrangement of membranes made of the same kind of oil molecules that form the cell's outer coat. If you observed the outer membrane as well as all the membranes inside the cell, you'd see various proteins and other substances carrying out the cell's inner life at a frantic pace. The external membrane is constantly forming little pouches and pockets in support of protein molecules (receptor sites) that receive messages from the outside world. And the inner membranes are also consumed with a dizzying set of activities. You would also notice that the activities of the cell proceed in waves, including, if you were to watch for twenty-four hours, a circadian rhythm.

The necessary speed of these transactions depends on the superflexibility of the membranes; if they are stiff, the cells' business simply can't take place at the proper rate. Therefore, the oils from which cell membranes are made also need to be extremely flexible. Thin oils work best.

THIN OILS MAKE THE MOST FLEXIBLE
CELL MEMBRANES

You can appreciate the difference between thin and thick oils simply by looking at the array of fats and oils found in every supermarket.

In the meat department there are animal fats that are basically white solid slabs at room temperature; they may melt in the heat of an oven but are still rather stiff at body temperature, which is their destiny after you eat them.

In the fish department are oils that are much more flexible. These are semifluid when the fish is swimming around in cold water; they liquefy at room temperature and become quite runny at human body temperature. Cold water fish, such as salmon, tuna, mackerel, bluefish, sardines, and herring, have the most liquid oils and are best for forming flexible cell membranes. (In fact, besides flaxseeds, these are the best food sources of omega-3 oils.)

FLAXSEED OIL

Flaxseed oil is an integral part of the Circadian Diet. The oil is extracted from the seeds of the flax plant, which is grown to make linen. Historically, in some parts of the world, especially eastern Europe, when the flax was harvested, the seeds were set aside to make oil. The process involved smashing the seeds with sufficient force to press out the oil, which was then kept for use in the kitchen and the medicine chest. It was used as a remedy for burns and to make dressings, since it made a good vehicle to carry medicinal substances into the skin.

Flaxseed oil consists of 40 percent alpha-linolenic acid; no other oil comes close to that concentration. It is so rich in ALA that taking a small amount of flaxseed oil every day is enough to give you the flexible cell membranes you need, as well as more manageable hair and skin and a reduction in your risk for many chronic illnesses. In your body, ALA is converted to eicosapentaenoic acid (EPA) and docosahexanoic acid (DHA), the same substances that are in cod liver oil or fish oil. If the chemical processes in your body are working well, flaxseed oil and fish oil are more or less interchangeable, although flaxseed oil provides the molecules that are best suited for making flexible cell membranes. However, if you are diabetic, alcoholic, nutritionally impaired, or very old, these processes may not be working well, in which case fish oil is the thing for you.

Next are the various types of vegetable—sometimes called salad or cooking—oils. You will find olive, corn, peanut, safflower, soy, sunflower, canola, and walnut oils. Of these, olive, canola, and walnut are the most flexible. Unfortunately, you will not find flaxseed oil, although it's the richest source of flexible oils; for that you'd have to go to the health food store.

REFINED VEGETABLE OILS LACK AN ESSENTIAL INGREDIENT

Before about 1950, the only commercially available fats for consumption were lard, butter, margarine, and olive oil. But thanks to new methods of extraction, oils made from cottonseed, corn, coconut, palm, soybeans, and sunflower and safflower seeds have made a sea change in the American diet. The process involves crushing the raw materials until they form an oily mash that is subjected to extraction using solvents similar to dry cleaning fluid. This procedure forces out much more oil than had been previously possible, making the venture commercially profitable.

These vegetable oils naturally contain a small amount of alpha-linolenic acid (ALA), as well as a large proportion of the omega-6 family of essential fatty acids, which are also important for health. However, the ALA—the most nutritionally valuable part of the oils—is intentionally removed so that they will have a long shelf life, because ALA is the fatty acid that goes rancid the most rapidly. This refining is not unlike what is done when sugar is refined from sugar cane or white flour is refined from whole wheat, other processes in which most of the nutritionally important parts of the grain are discarded and the starchy white remains are offered to us as food.

In addition, many of these oils have also undergone hydrogenation, creating misshapen, stiffened trans fats in the process. Along with the saturated fats typically found in animal products such as butter, trans fats have been linked to heart disease.

Refined oils are problematic because when it comes to fat, you are what you eat. Although the body can manufacture fat molecules (for example, from sugar), it generally doesn't bother to do so. Instead, it uses the fat molecules you eat, which pass relatively unaltered into the fat reserves of your body. Quite literally, all foods that you eat, except fat, go through a violent process of destruction as they are chewed, delivered to your stomach and small intestine, digested, and sent to your liver to be checked for toxins and go through final processing. This process breaks the food molecules down into relatively neutral small parts that can then be re-assembled and sent into your bloodstream or burned for fuel.

But the fats you eat bypass the liver altogether. Instead, fat moves from your intestine directly into special vessels called lymph ducts. These join one big lymph duct that passes right up the middle of your chest and empties into the bloodstream at a large vein under your left collarbone. Thus, the transfer of fat from food into the blood is remarkably direct. This is evident as a milky appearance of the usually clear amber serum in blood drawn from someone who has eaten a regular meal containing any amount of fat and certainly after a particularly fatty meal. An analysis of the particular kinds of oil molecules in the blood will exhibit the charac-teristic pattern of their sources and reveal what the proportion and kinds of fat in the person's diet have been.

If you expect that the only thing you are going to do with oil when you get it into your bloodstream is turn it into fat, then you may not care whether it came from fish, beef, or olives. But if you want to use the raw materials in the fat for making healthy cell membranes, it matters a lot.

FATS, HORMONES, AND INFLAMMATION

Besides the need for flexible oils to make flexible cell membranes, the kinds of oils you eat matter for other reasons. First, omega-3 and omega-6 fatty acids are the raw materials your body uses for making prostaglandin hormones. (Originally named for the prostate gland from which they were first isolated, it turns out they have nothing exclusively to do with the prostate gland.) They are now recognized as one of the main vehicles for cell-to-cell communication throughout the body. That this communica-tion plays a role in the proper working of the reproductive system becomes evident when some women experience improved reproductive function, such as a resumption of menstrual periods, after consuming a supplement of flaxseed oil.

Second, given the role of inflammation in almost every kind of chronic illness, including cardiovascular disease, the anti-inflammatory effects of omega-3 oils explain another of their benefits. Omega-3 oils are natural blockers of the bad messengers (arachidonic acid and its children) that are the key to the body's production of the heat, swelling, redness, and pain that we call inflammation.

Running short on omega-3 oils has a profound effect on your body's health. Yet it's likely that you're not consuming enough; omega-3 deficiency is at epidemic levels in this country. Scientists think that the optimal diet should contain a *balanced* ratio of omega-6 fatty acids to omega-3 fatty acids; the typical American diet is between 14 to 1 and 20 to 1.[2] There's also an issue of dietary balance. Although we all need to eat some omega-6 fatty acids, a diet too high in omega-6 oils interferes with the metabolism of omega-3 oils.

SIGNALS OF OMEGA-3 DEFICIENCY: HAIR, SKIN, AND NAILS

Problems with hair, skin, and nails often come down to the fats and oils in your diet. Eating—or not eating—certain oils, particularly flaxseed oil and others that contain omega-3 fatty acids, can make an enormous difference.

On television, I often see advertisements where an attractive model tosses her head so as to make her hair swing gracefully through the air; if her hair didn't swing, the head toss really wouldn't be worth it, would it? After all, if you toss your head and your hair doesn't swing but simply sticks out of your scalp like the straw coming out of a scarecrow's sleeve, the whole effect is lost.

What the advertisement is trying to show you, however silly and misleading it may be, is that your hair should be silky and have a certain texture, flexibility, and obedience. In other words, it should be "manageable." The model has used a chemical treatment to make her hair manageable. But there is another way to get your hair to oblige without resorting to an arsenal of chemical ammunition.

I wager that billions of dollars are being spent on hair management in the United States. If the people who stock their showers with various shampoos, gels, mousses and conditioners invested in eating healthy oils it would cost a mere fraction of the amount they spend on hair care products. And even as they conquered lackluster hair and split ends, they'd reap the dividend of a lowered risk for cancer and other chronic health problems.

The same is true for fingernails. Having lived in parts of the world where people decorate—or, depending on your point of view, mutilate—their bodies in various ways that have some esthetic purpose, it's not for me to weigh in too heavily against nail decoration. Before women come in to my office, though, I routinely ask them to refrain from wearing nail polish so that I can look at their fingernails, which are an expression of their general health. Fingernails also provide clues of mineral deficiencies (little white spots or flecks) or other nutritional problems. Some women

---

TREATING OMEGA-3 OIL DEFICIENCY

I regularly see patients whose health and appearance are transformed by supplements of flaxseed oil. If you have marked symptoms of omega-3 oil deficiency, especially of your hair, skin, or nails, try taking 1 to 2 teaspoons of flaxseed oil in addition to the shake (or you can put it in the shake) for a few months. Buy only expeller-pressed flaxseed oil in an opaque bottle; make sure you check the expiration date, and be sure to keep it in the refrigerator.

You may substitute fish oils in the form of cod liver oil, or a more modern version of cod liver oil in pill form called MaxEPA, if you are one of the few people with whom flaxseed oil doesn't agree. You'll know you have a problem with flaxseed oil if you develop a rash, digestive complaints, or any other symptom that starts when you take it and goes away when you stop.

Unless you are one of the few people with an allergy to flaxseed, there is no harm in taking the amounts that I am recommending. But I caution you not to get the idea that if a little bit of flaxseed powder or oil is good, more must be better. Consuming large quantities won't do you any extra good, and it might do you some harm. Dr. Donald O. Rudin, the pioneer of the chemistry and clinical use of omega-3 oils, successfully used daily doses of 3 ounces of flaxseed oil in treating patients, so I don't think you have to be terribly cautious about short-term experiments with large amounts of flaxseed oil provided you experience no negative symptoms.[3] However, large amounts of ground flaxseeds can be mischievous, and you should never eat more than 3 tablespoons per day, because it could interfere with your thyroid function. Remember, a little bit goes a long way.

misunderstand my instructions and, instead of painting their nails, come in wearing plastic nails, because their own fingernails simply won't grow. Growing healthy fingernails seems fundamental to me; with a few very rare exceptions, there is no such thing as going bald in the nails. Nails that crack, split, are brittle and break easily, or just plain won't grow are signs of omega-3 oil deficiency.

There is one more area where oil questions really come into play. Hair and nails are part of the general department of the body doctors call the integument, that is, the coverings. A major part of the integument is your skin. Acne, dull skin, greasy skin, dry skin, the greasy and dry skin called combination skin in television advertisements about a decade or two ago, patchy dullness on your cheeks, dandruff, seborrhea, psoriasis, chicken skin (little bumps on the back of the arms), alligator skin (usually found on the lower legs where the skin gets a cracked dry appearance), and cracking skin of the fingertips, which is usually worse or sometimes happens only in winter, are all signs that you need your oil changed.

MORE THAN SKIN DEEP

The payoff for consuming the right oils isn't only skin deep; it can affect your physical and mental well-being in many ways. And besides feeling generally well in the short term, the benefits you get from eating the right fats include a lower risk of cancer and other chronic illnesses.

The diagnosis and treatment of complex chronic illness often requires an extensive dialog with my patients, physical and laboratory examinations, and several attempts at tailoring to get it right, even when it is ultimately successful. Sometimes, however, and fairly often in the realm of fatty acid problems, heeding simple clues can lead to quick fixes.

Helen dropped into my office several years ago to visit her sister Sue, who was a medical student working with me at the time. Because she had been hearing stories from me and my patients about the remarkable effects of consuming flaxseed oil, especially with regard to skin, nail, and hair symptoms, Sue wondered if her sister's skin condition might be a clue that she would benefit from taking a supplement of flaxseed oil.

What Helen had was not what you would even call a rash; it was a raised ridge or a faint waxy pink line drawn across the V of her upper chest. Technically speaking, it was an unusual expression of seborrhea, which is in the dandruff spectrum, but she didn't actually have dandruff. The rash had responded to the cortisone cream that a dermatologist gave her, but of course the cortisone didn't make the rash go away; it just suppressed it as long as she was using the cream.

Helen's other problems included a profound depression that had been going on for four to five years, the same duration as the rash. She was working with a psychiatrist, but the drugs then in use—this was before the days of Prozac—were not helpful. In addition, she had not gotten her period for two or three years. By taking progesterone for a few days each month she could be induced to have a period, but on her own she failed.

Breaking the rules that apply to doctors who are asked to do curbside consultations, especially for people who have been more or less dragged into your office by a relative, I nevertheless suggested that she take a supplement of a tablespoon of flaxseed oil once a day for a month or two. In a month's time her period resumed, her depression lifted completely, and her skin became entirely normal.

You may be skeptical that consuming omega-3 oils can improve everything from skin problems to depression. However, because fats work at the cellular level, a deficiency in fatty acids may express itself in many ways: irregular periods, a skin rash, depression, rheumatoid arthritis, or

---

PURSLANE: THE OMEGA-3 POWERHOUSE OF THE FUTURE

Most gardeners will tell you that purslane is a weed. But this low, creeping plant with green fleshy leaves and purple-tinted stems, long eaten in some Mediterranean, eastern European, and Asian countries, may soon be cultivated more often than it is pulled out. In fact, breeders have developed domesticated purslanes that grow taller and more upright than their wild cousin; these new varieties are available in a number of seed catalogs.

Purslane is full of omega-3 fatty acids—in fact, it's one of the richest sources in the plant world—as well as a host of antioxidants, including vitamins C and E, beta-carotene, and glutathione. Its lemony flavor makes purslane a fine addition to salads. It can also be steamed, stir-fried, or puréed.

any one of a number of inflammatory or autoimmune problems such as psoriasis, asthma, colitis, allergies, and Crohn's disease.

Illness can be triggered or expressed in highly individual ways from one person to another. But we all share common features in the landscape of our biochemistry that make it easier to understand how these fatty acids give you more manageable hair and clearer skin as well as improve the functions of the hearts, lungs, intestines, and reproductive system. Whether or not you have signs of deficiency, adding omega-3 oils to your diet is an important step to well-being.

24:00
25:00
01:00
02:00
03:00
04:00
05:00
06:00
07:00
08:00
09:00
10:00
11:00
12:00
13:00
14:00
15:00
16:00
17:00
18:00
19:00
20:00
21:00
22:00
23:00
24:00
25:00
01:00

CHAPTER

8

Intestinal Flora:
Small Creatures Alter Big Rhythms

Margaret Simons had been in perfect health all of her life. Then, at the age of 41, after a virus and severe laryngitis that had dragged on for several weeks, a doctor put her on antibiotics, and things began to go downhill. She felt spacey and experienced tightness in the chest and an upset, bloated stomach and loose stools; she also began to lose weight. The doctor put her on a second three-week course of antibiotics and, when she still wasn't feeling better, started her on a third course.

By the time she came to me, three years later, she'd been to many specialists. Although she looked fine—as if she were all set to go out and play tennis—she had a list of problems as long as my arm. She had a vaginal yeast infection and had developed multiple food allergies, for which she was on a "caveman diet," eating only meat, chicken, fish, and occasionally potato. After the deaths of her parents, for whom she'd been the primary caregiver, Margaret had reached a low point. She collapsed with a high fever and bad chills and was diagnosed with chronic fatigue syndrome.

She began to feel better after I treated her yeast infection (and presumed intestinal yeast overgrowth) with Diflucan, an antifungal medication, and she has continued to gradually recover as we've tried many different treatments. Her chronic fatigue is gone, and her energy has returned. But her difficulties with many foods, especially carbohydrates, remain.

What happened to Margaret is far from unusual. The antibiotics damaged her intestinal flora, and now she has a chronic yeast problem:

She doesn't completely digest her food, which ferments and causes her yeast overgrowth to flare up periodically with dramatic consequences.

WHAT ARE INTESTINAL FLORA?

Your flora consist of one quadrillion individual germs that inhabit your body. This collection of germs exists on your skin, the surface of your eyes, in your digestive tract—from your mouth all the way to the other end—and, if you are a woman, in your vagina.

The germs that inhabit your digestive tract and other surfaces of your body are collectively like a single organ with an intricate task: to do biochemical feats of extraordinary complexity that you cannot do for yourself. These germs carry out chemical transformations, including the synthesis of vitamins and other nutrients, that are vital for your health. They play a crucial role in the translation of the information contained in your food into messages that your body can understand.

Although these germs are life forms that existed on our planet for literally hundreds of millions of years before the arrival of human beings, your flora are usually a friendly presence inside your body. On the Circadian Diet, where you are consuming most carbohydrates in the evenings, the digestion of these carbohydrates with the help of healthy intestinal flora will promote sleep and supply your body with the raw materials it needs during the night. And your intestinal flora will convert the soy protein, flaxseed powder, and rye fiber you eat into protective substances that help regulate your hormone chemistry and reduce your risk of cancer. In short, your flora help you to get all the rhythmic benefits of the diet.

But the wrong kind of flora can produce toxins that interfere with your chemistry, undermine your health, and deprive you of the benefits of the Circadian Diet. Modern technology allows us to understand that undesirable intestinal bacteria and yeasts have a chemical warfare arsenal, including substances that mimic neurotransmitters or key players in carbohydrate metabolism. When they find their way into the bloodstream they masquerade as your own molecules, provoking serious problems.[1]

ANTIBIOTICS DAMAGE FLORA

Often patients worry about liver damage when I prescribe certain medications. Their concern is justified. Medications frequently do bother the liver, which is the body's main detoxification organ and therefore subject to damage when overloaded by substances that are toxic or that for some reason the liver perceives as toxic. Generally speaking, though, your liver is an extremely robust organ with amazing powers of recovery following injury.

In contrast, your flora is a rather delicate "organ," which can be significantly and enduringly injured by even a single dose of an antibiotic. Once damaged, it can take months, if not years, to heal, even if you take special action to ensure its recovery. So the first question you should ask whenever the subject of certain medications, especially antibiotics, comes up is: "What can be done to protect my flora?"

Damage to your intestinal germ population is the universal consequence of taking antibiotics. Every time you take an antibiotic, even the smallest dose, you damage your flora just as if you burned your finger in a flame or stubbed your toe. The difference is that you may feel no pain, even though the injury is much worse and more enduring. If you don't feel well after taking an antibiotic, it is almost certainly because of the damage to your flora, but the ways in which you feel badly may or may not include your digestive tract and may vary greatly from person to person.

Antibiotics kill the good germs as well as the bacteria that are their intended target. Without the action of good germs to convert components of soy, rye, and flaxseed into hormonally beneficial substances, you may be deprived of their cancer-preventing effects, for months and possibly longer. Meanwhile, bad germs multiply in your digestive tract, altering your hormone chemistry and causing mischief that's associated with increased risk of breast cancer in women and prostate cancer in men. In addition, release of toxins from these bad germs can cause certain types of arthritis, interfere with your body's detoxification systems, and slyly mimic molecules involved in your carbohydrate and neurotransmitter chemistry.

I'm not trying to discourage you from taking an antibiotic if you need one for the treatment of a confirmed infection. Sometimes, however, when there is no clear-cut evidence of a bacterial infection, a course of antibiotics becomes a judgment call. Under these circumstances, many people are inclined to ask for an antibiotic because they believe it will help them feel better sooner. I urge you to think twice if you find yourself in this situation.

PREVENTING THE DAMAGE FROM ANTIBIOTICS

If you have to take an antibiotic, there are things you can do to prevent damage to your flora. It's important to eat plenty of fiber. Germs like to feed on fiber; without generous amounts of it, your flora will have a hard time regaining their balance. Whole grain rye bread is an excellent choice because it contains the rye fiber that is especially rich in good lignans. Barley is another good source of lignans. Leafy vegetables are fiber-rich and, of course, flaxseed fiber, which is included in the Rhythmic Shake, is especially rich in substances that feed flora.

Yogurt, a key ingredient in the Rhythmic Shake, contains beneficial germs such as acidophilus, which play a crucial role in suppressing yeasts and other harmful organisms. (Be sure you use yogurt that contains *live* cultures.) You should also take a supplement, in the form of a pill, containing large and varied amounts of normal bowel flora. Many brands are available, although the quality and quantity of the germs included in flora replacement remedies varies. It's best to stick with well-established brand names, like Klaire Laboratories (Vital Life), Metagenics, and Allergy Research. Look for formulas that contain acidophilus (lactobacillus), bifidus, and lateroflora. Products containing inulin (in which Jerusalem artichokes are especially rich), fructooligosaccharides (an ingredient in UltraClear products), and glutamine are also helpful in restoring normal flora and healing the gut.

YEAST OVERGROWTH INTERFERES WITH
CARBOHYDRATE CHEMISTRY

Unfortunately, you can't always prevent damage to your flora. It's especially important to be vigilant for symptoms of an overgrowth of bad yeast germs, which are the most likely to multiply following a course of an antibiotic. The potential consequences of their long-term residence in your digestive tract may be severe. Symptoms to watch for include:

- Recurrent vaginitis

- Bloating, gas, digestive discomfort

- Constipation, diarrhea, or change in bowel habits or in stool odor or color

- Difficulty concentrating or a feeling of spaciness

- Short-term memory problems

- Fatigue

- Depression

- Fluid retention

- Signs of inflammation such as muscle or joint pain

- Skin rashes

- Wheezing, sneezing, or stuffiness

- Urinary symptoms

Apart from the obvious symptoms caused by their overgrowth, yeast germs can produce a quieter sort of mischief by disrupting your carbohydrate chemistry. This is one reason why some individuals have a harder time properly handling carbohydrates than others. The uncontrolled growth of yeast germs interferes with the Circadian Diet.

Yeasts, along with other fungi, are classified as neither animal nor vegetable. We know fungi principally as the mushrooms we buy in the vegetable section at the market, but fungi are very un-vegetablelike. Vegetables are plants; they use the sun's energy directly and combine carbon dioxide and water to make carbohydrates. Yeasts and other fungi are more like animals; they consume carbohydrates to recover the sun's energy by taking sugar molecules apart, just as we do.

Some eight to ten thousand years ago, one of our ancestors figured out that if you tightly covered a container of grape juice, it would turn to wine. The germ that ferments wine is a yeast that grows naturally on the surface of the grape. Nowadays winemakers introduce a particular strain of yeast that has been selected because of its especially good winemaking properties, but you can still produce wine from the naturally occurring germs that live on the surface of a healthy grape and account for the whitish coating that you see on unwashed grapes. Fermentation of grape juice—the breakdown of the sugar in the grapes by germs to form carbon dioxide, water, alcohol, and vinegar—allowed the juice to be saved for future consumption; otherwise it would have spoiled. The details of carbohydrate chemistry were first figured out in the brewing industry as scientists investigated the chemical workings of the fungus responsible for this fermentation. The carbohydrate chemistry worked out by these first biochemists is about the same for all living things, from bacteria to human beings.

Unfortunately, yeast and other fungi are the masters of carbohydrate chemistry. They are low-life, low-light creatures that are able to extract the last traces of light stored in once living materials as they decay. And yeast germs are remarkably like human body cells. They have the same kind of complicated innards, including mitochondria, a nucleus, and various apparatus in the water surrounding the nucleus. Yeasts also have a circadian rhythm, but the timing of that rhythm in the yeasts in people's innards has never been determined. Yeasts can make substances called analog inhibitors that confuse your body and disturb the way it normally breaks down cellulose, starches, and sugars. They interfere with your ability to extract and use the energy stored in carbohydrates that is so vital to your body's nighttime tasks of repair, healing, and detoxification.

TREATING YEAST OVERGROWTH

If you have signs of yeast overgrowth, you may need professional advice from a physician experienced in treating people with this problem. Unfortunately, the majority of physicians in the United States have been slow to recognize that changes in flora wrought by antibiotics disturb hormone chemistry or affect overall health.

A physician or other medical professional licensed to prescribe drugs can help you obtain an antifungal medicine. Prescription medicines include Nystatin, which is utterly safe, or Diflucan, Sporanox, Lamisil, or Nizoral, each of which has a tiny risk associated with it. All are effective at killing yeasts that have grown up as a result of antibiotics. But like the antibiotics that are used to kill bacteria, the effectiveness of these antifungal medications hinges on the particular yeast germ in question. No one antifungal is better than the others unless one considers the possible sensitivity and resistance of the targeted germ. If you prefer natural remedies for yeast overgrowth, your choices include citrus seed extract, garlic, oregano oil, goldenseal, and other herbal remedies. Other useful over-the-counter pharmaceuticals are caprylic acid and undecylenic acid.

If you have a yeast overgrowth, you should follow the Circadian Diet strictly and carefully limit most of your carbohydrates to the evening. In addition, you should avoid some foods entirely. It's especially important to stay away from refined flours and sugars, including honey, maple sugar, molasses, and corn sweeteners, which all tend to feed yeasts. Fruits and fruit juices, no matter how healthy they are otherwise, are sugary and should be avoided. Fruits are also problematic because their surfaces are normally covered with yeasts. These yeasts are not an infectious threat. Rather they irritate your immune system, which is already engaged in an ongoing fight with yeast germs, to the point where you may develop an allergy to yeasts and their various cousins in the world of molds. You should also refrain from consuming foods or beverages that are fermented, brewed, or leavened, like breads, wine, beer, vinegar, and most crackers. An exception to this rule is yogurt, which is a product of fermentation produced by lactobacillus, a friendly germ whose growth you want to encourage. (For a more detailed discussion of yeast-free diets, see my Web site: www: sbakermd.com/info/yeast/yeast1htm, *The Yeast Connection,* by William G. Crook, or *The Missing Diagnosis,* by C. Orian Truss.)[2]

If you feel better after taking these steps, then you don't need to do anything more, apart from staying vigilant for signs of a recurrence. You've licked your yeast problem, and you can continue the Circadian Diet with the knowledge that you are now receiving all of its benefits. Try reintroducing yeasty foods, and let your body tell you if and when you regain some degree of tolerance.

If you are still ill, something other than yeast overgrowth may be causing damage to your flora. There are laboratory tests to assess this, but they are imperfect. Good tests to measure urine or blood levels of the hormone modulators that the germs of your digestive tract produce from the isoflavones and lignans in your food are not yet available, although I believe they will be soon, as doctors become more aware of the negative consequences of taking antibiotics. For now, the best test is a Comprehensive Digestive Stool Analysis (CDSA), done at Great Smokies Laboratory in Asheville, North Carolina. This test measures many aspects of digestive flora and function.

FEEDING YOUR DIGESTIVE TRACT

Butyrate, a fatty acid manufactured from food fiber by intestinal germ populations, is one important aspect of digestive function measured by the CDSA. Its functions are well documented, but most laboratories don't yet have a test for it. Butyrate is and will be of compelling interest as research continues on the interaction between bowel flora and nutrition.

The cells that line the digestive tract of your body form a huge surface, about the size of a tennis court. The care and feeding of this enormous membrane is critical to your health because it is on this membrane that you transact business with the outside world. Here you allow in what you need for your nutrition, and at the same time you keep out toxins or other materials that don't belong in your bloodstream. It's a major feat, especially when you consider that this membrane is only the thickness of your eyelid. And it's crucial to your health; when inappropriate materials get into your bloodstream it can lead to food allergies, depression of your immune system, and other serious problems.

These important cells lining your digestive tract are constantly exposed to food that is tumbling along the passageway. Just like all cells in the body, they need nourishment. Are they eating any of this food directly, or do they wait for the nutrients in your food to be absorbed into your bloodstream and sent back to them, just like the cells in your liver, brain, muscles, or other organs? Is there a different mechanism for feeding the cells that happen to live on the lining of the digestive tract or, so to speak, on the riverbank? And why does this matter, anyway?

As it turns out, nature does allow the cells of the digestive tract to eat food directly from the river on whose banks they live. In the upper digestive tract this food comes in the form of an amino acid called glutamine; in the lower digestive tract the food is butyrate, with some help from two other fatty acids, acetate and propionate.

Butyrate is digested from fiber in your food by normal digestive flora. When your flora is disturbed, you are less able to convert fiber into butyrate to feed your gut lining, which is then less able to protect you from absorbing unwanted materials into your bloodstream. People with low stool butyrate levels run a higher risk of developing bowel cancer.[3] When you hear people say that fiber isn't important, remember that fiber feeds the flora that in turn feeds the lining of your digestive tract, which allows you to absorb phytonutrients.

The role of healthy intestinal flora in converting certain critical phytonutrients into effective protection against cancer, heart disease, osteoporosis, inflammatory diseases, and other serious chronic illnesses justifies your concern about its care and feeding. Your flora are crucial to your health in numerous ways and play an indispensable role in allowing you to get the value from the fiber and protein in the Circadian Diet.

25:00
24:00
25:00
01:00
02:00
03:00
04:00
05:00
06:00
07:00
08:00
09:00
10:00
11:00
12:00
13:00
14:00
15:00
16:00
17:00
18:00
19:00
20:00
21:00
22:00
23:00
24:00
25:00
01:00

CHAPTER

9

Drugs and Supplements

F our prosperous friends from Denver—Joel, Dennis, Eva, and Veronica—were taking a trip to Italy. They planned to fly to Rome, rent a car, drive to Sorrento, and then go back to Rome. Veronica, who knew of my friendship with Charles Ehret, the author of *Overcoming Jet Lag,* asked me how they might best prepare for the eight-hour time difference between Denver and Rome so they'd lose as little time as possible once they arrived in Italy.[1] (See the appendix for more details on how to beat jet lag with diet.)

Here's how they did it. They each followed a different path to overcoming the negative effects of crossing numerous time zones in a short period. Maybe you can guess how each one fared.

Veronica, a neurosurgeon, passed on my advice to the others yet ignored it herself. Instead, she followed her hard-working doctor's pattern of pushing herself, working until 2:00 a.m. the night before the trip, which was to begin the next evening. The day of the trip she got up early to make rounds at the hospital and rushed home to finish some errands and pack. On her way home, she stopped for fast food because she had skipped breakfast.

Settling into the first class cabin on the airplane, Veronica gladly accepted the flight attendant's offer of champagne and replenished her glass four times before takeoff. She took one refill of her predinner cocktail and was sampling a third wine selection on the menu when she dozed off. Two hours later she awakened, ate dinner, and then stayed up to watch the movie with Eva. She dozed again until an hour before arrival in Rome, where she woke herself up with coffee. In the afternoon, she walked all over Sorrento and had a big fish dinner, wine, and an espresso. After taking a sleeping pill, she went to bed at 11:00 p.m., waking up to a big breakfast of three eggs and sausage.

Although Eva, an actress, didn't follow my advice either, she approached the day of departure well rested. She had a big breakfast and went to the hairdresser. On the airplane, she ate a large first-class dinner without coffee or alcohol, stayed up for the movie, and then read a book until she dozed off. Once in Italy, she had two cups of espresso with bread and jam for breakfast, dozed in the car on the way to Sorrento, and went straight to bed when they arrived at the hotel. She got up for a dinner of fish and pasta and went back to sleep at midnight Sorrento time (4:00 p.m. in Denver). After a restless night, she woke up to a breakfast of coffee, bread, and jam.

Dennis, an artist, took my recommendations seriously and prepared by going almost entirely without food on the day of departure. The previous day he had eaten heavily; the day before that he had eaten sparsely; the day before that he had eaten heavily. So his pattern had been feast, fast, feast, fast. On the plane, he did not partake of the luxurious first-class fare and freely flowing champagne, cocktails, and wine. Instead, he ate a light meal followed by three cups of strong black coffee. He put on a mask to shut out the light, snoozed intermittently through the buzz engendered by the coffee, and finally took half of a mild sedative to help him sleep. When the flight attendant woke him at 2:00 a.m. Denver time, which was 10:00 a.m. in Italy, he ate a large breakfast of eggs, sausage, and one piece of toast, with no jam, juice, or coffee. He stayed up all day, except for a forty-five-minute nap, and had a large dinner of pasta with a big dessert and no coffee. At 10:00 p.m. he took ½ milligram of melatonin, and he went to bed at midnight.

Joel, a lawyer who avoided extremes, was well rested and ate moderately on the day of departure. On the plane, he had a cocktail and one glass of wine with dinner, turning down the coffee so he could get some sleep. He managed to doze, then enjoyed a breakfast of coffee and bread, sweet rolls, and jam. He took on the job of driving to Sorrento, where he went sightseeing. Exhausted, he went back to the hotel and took a three-hour nap, waking up for a dinner of fish and pasta. He went to bed at

2:00 a.m., or 6:00 p.m. Denver time. A summary of the travelers' activities appears in the table.

FOUR-PERSON JET LAG COMPARISON

	VERONICA	EVA	DENNIS	JOEL
Before departure	Little sleep	Well rested	Ate heavily. On previous days alternated feasting and fasting	Well rested
Day of departure	Skipped breakfast, rushed around and ate a lot	Big breakfast	Very little food	Ate moderately
On the plane	Got drunk, ate a lot, stayed up for the movie	Large meal, no coffee or alcohol, slept	Light meal, three cups of strong black coffee, mask, mild sedative, slept	Cocktail and wine with moderate dinner, no coffee, dozed
Breakfast in Rome	Coffee	Two espressos, bread and jam	Eggs, sausage, one toast, no coffee	Coffee and bread, sweet rolls, jam
Day in Sorrento	Walked all over	Slept in car, to bed on arrival at hotel	45-minute nap, walked around	Sightseeing, then three-hour nap
Evening in Sorrento	Big fish dinner, wine, espresso	Fish and pasta	Pasta and big dessert, no coffee	Fish and pasta
Night in Sorrento	Sleeping pill, bed at 11:00 p.m.	Bed at midnight, poor sleep	Melatonin at 10:00 p.m., bed at midnight	Bed at 1:00 a.m.
Breakfast	Three eggs and sausage	Coffee, bread, and jam	Eggs, sausage, one toast, no coffee	Coffee, bread, and jam

Each of the friends fared differently. On the day of arrival, Dennis was in the best shape, and Veronica had a headache from the champagne but was otherwise alert. By the following day both of them were fine. But Joel and Eva took several days to recover from the fatigue, difficulty concentrating, constipation, irritability, and general lack of enthusiasm for traipsing around to see the sights that people endure when they are suffering from jet lag.

Dennis and Veronica did well for opposite reasons. Dennis's case is fairly straightforward. He strictly followed the jet lag diet program, so his body became "entrained" by the alternating days of feasting and fasting, (or eating very lightly). In addition, he was more sensitive to the effects of caffeine when taken after fasting on the day of departure. The coffee he drank at night on the plane helped reset his body clock in the direction that was appropriate for eastbound travel. At breakfast Italian time, Dennis ate a high protein breakfast without coffee. The protein nudged his body toward a morning rhythm; he avoided coffee so as not to interfere with his body clock. He stayed up all day, napping for less than forty-five minutes, and had a high carbohydrate dinner, again pushing his body toward Sorrento time, which was evening. He capped everything off by taking a small dose of melatonin. Because he maximized his chances for rapidly resetting his body clock, he felt well by the following day, although there would still be a lag of physiologic measurements, such as body temperature, during the ensuing few days as he adjusted to Italian time.

In contrast, Veronica broke most of the rules. She got into a state of exhaustion over last-minute preparations, ate heavily during the day before she got on the plane, and then proceeded to get drunk. When one would normally be asleep, Italian time, she stayed up to watch the movie. (Remember, Dennis was protecting his eyes from light and minimizing any social stimulation.) She had coffee on the plane as well as at breakfast, then stayed up all day walking in Sorrento. She finished her day with a large, high protein dinner, more wine, and coffee, followed by a sedative.

Still, except for a slight hangover, Veronica felt all right the next day. Her excessive consumption of caffeine and alcohol, as well as the sedative, had temporarily erased her circadian rhythm: in Sorrento, her body was not on Denver time; it was on no time at all. Paradoxically, she was able to get onto Sorrento time more quickly because she was starting from scratch, having caused such massive disruption of her day and night cycle.

Eva was well rested and therefore likely to have a strong, well-established circadian rhythm when she left Denver; this actually worked against her when it came to re-establishing her settings for Italy. Several other mistakes compounded the problem. She stayed up for the movie and read a book when, on Italian time, she should have been sleeping. Her morning coffee pushed her clock in a westward rather than an eastward direction. And by taking a nap lasting more than forty-five minutes when they arrived in Sorrento she gave her body too much of a "time to sleep" signal and deprived herself of the exposure to sunlight that would have helped reset her clock to Italian time.

Joel, being a man of moderation, did nothing drastic one way or another to prepare for the time change. He didn't help his body adjust to the new time and, like Eva, by taking a long nap on the day of arrival actually inhibited his body's capacity to get the appropriate signals for resetting its clock.

Circadian Rhythm Is Flexible

The experiences of Veronica, Eva, Joel, and Dennis illustrate two messages that are significant for the Circadian Prescription. One is that caffeine and alcohol are drugs that strongly affect circadian rhythms. In moderation, caffeine tends to reset your body clock backward when taken in the morning and forward when taken in the evening. It has a neutral effect when you drink it at 4:00 p.m., or what might be considered teatime in England. And drinking alcohol to excess, especially late in the evening, simply knocks out your circadian rhythm.

The second message is that it's possible to reset your body clock or to disrupt it, depending on how you go about it. Human circadian rhythm is flexible, but it takes a concerted effort to exploit its adaptability. Protein and carbohydrate, light and dark, activity and rest, and drugs are all time-givers that play roles in orchestrating the daily adjustment of your built-in circadian rhythm of more than twenty-four-hours to the twenty-four-hour cycle of our planet. But your body's circadian flexibility works two ways. On the one hand, these multiple timegivers are quite dependable in resetting your body clock to twenty-four hours. But if the timegivers are powerful enough to reset your circadian rhythm by an hour every day, they are also strong enough to work against you as well as for you; their powerful effects, if ill timed, can be negative.

Daily exposure to natural light is a strong timegiver. It's always a good idea to follow the rules about exposure to light. Whenever possible, get out into the sun during the day and be sure to protect yourself from light at night. (On the plane, Joel's mask may have looked weird, but he was actually right on target by trying to completely avoid nighttime exposure to light.) Since most of us simply do not or cannot be outdoors every day and stay in utter darkness at night, the relative influence of the timegivers relating to food and activity is even stronger. If you work indoors and are not exposed to natural light on a regular basis, your control over what you eat and when you eat it, especially the timing of protein and carbohydrates, becomes relatively more important in reinforcing a strong circadian rhythm.

Some of the steps you can take to improve your situation are counterintuitive, like the Circadian Diet, where you switch from the typical high carbohydrate breakfast to one that emphasizes protein. In fact, we often do things in ways that run counter to supporting and taking advantage of circadian rhythm. Let's say you have an exam on Wednesday and another at 9:00 a.m. on Friday morning. You have forty-eight hours in which to cram, eat, sleep, and worry. You figure that in preparing for Friday's exam the best thing to do is to study at night when things are quiet and no one will bother you. So you drink a lot of coffee and stay up late on Wednesday and Thursday. You also sleep late on Thursday morning so that you are asleep at 9:00 a.m., twenty-four hours before your exam.

You've done it all wrong. Remember, excess caffeine will wipe out your circadian rhythm. And drinking moderate amounts of coffee and staying up all night is going to shift your circadian rhythm so that your body will end up thinking you're taking the exam in another time zone. Besides, it's best to prepare for the exam at the time of day when mental alertness is at its peak, which is in the morning (fortunately, that's also when you'll be taking the exam). A good night's sleep before a test is probably more important than an extra hour or two of cramming, so an early bedtime with a high carbohydrate dinner and no caffeine will help you not only sleep but sleep well. A high protein breakfast on Thursday and Friday before the exam will give you a strong energy boost. And studying on Thursday morning instead of sleeping late will give you the advantage of facing the exam when your body is used to studying. Once you've prepared in this way, if you feel that a strong cup of coffee just before the exam will help you sharpen your mind, I don't see much wrong with it. The short-term stimulant effect of coffee and its circadian consequences are sufficiently separated so that the caffeine you drink in the morning won't influence your circadian rhythm until the afternoon, when you won't care what time zone you're in.

Whether you are flying across time zones, taking an exam, or just going through the routines of your daily life, your body's flexibility allows the timegivers to reset your clock every day to the twenty-four-hour cycle of the planet. And if you become ill or if you stress your body, especially with shift work or jet travel, it's especially important to do whatever you can to support healthy circadian rhythm. (For more information about coping with the stresses of shift work, see the appendix.)

DRUGS THAT DESTROY OR REINFORCE CIRCADIAN RHYTHM

Drugs can also powerfully affect your circadian rhythm. Let's start with an example of something that, like alcohol or excess caffeine, tends to destroy circadian rhythm. Strong sedatives or sleeping pills, in medical parlance "hypnotics," do not produce real sleep. Nor do they favor the normal chemistry of sleep, which depends on a rising nighttime level of the neurotransmitter serotonin. They may be helpful for short-term use. Taken occasionally, they do not interfere too much with your functioning the following day. However, regular use of sleeping pills tends to deprive you of real sleep and to interfere with your circadian rhythm.

If you are following the Circadian Prescription to strengthen your circadian health and you have sleep problems, you may wish to consider taking tryptophan in the evening. This amino acid is the raw material from which your body normally makes its nighttime serotonin supply. The sleep it produces is different from what's achieved by sedatives, including

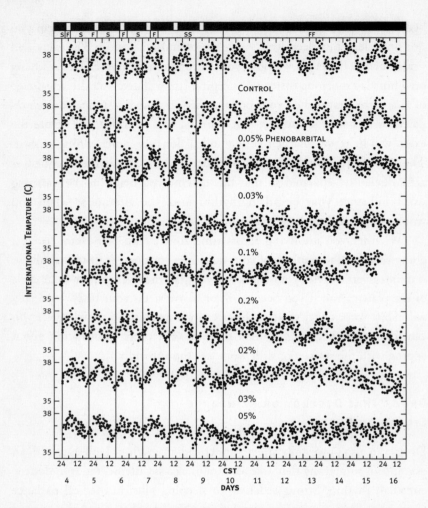

This experiment by Dr. Charles Ehret shows the effect of increasing doses of phenobarbital (a sleeping-pill type of medication) on the circadian rhythm of rats. Each dot represents a determination of the temperature of the rats, which rises and falls normally during each of the nine days before the drug is administered. The top series shows that the control animals, who receive no drug, continue to show the temperature ups and downs of a normal circadian rhythm. Each subsequent series below shows the effects of an increasing dose of the drug, which leads to the complete disorganization of the circadian rhythm, shown in the bottom series.

heavy-duty sleeping pills, because it reinforces the normal peak of serotonin at night, therefore supporting natural sleep and reinforcing healthy circadian rhythm. Consumed in doses of 500 to 1,000 milligrams with a carbohydrate snack in the evening, tryptophan has proved effective in promoting sleep in many people. You should not normally take tryptophan in the morning, except under professional advice for treatment of a problem other than sleep.

You may have difficulty obtaining tryptophan. It is now available only with a doctor's prescription because of a Food and Drug Administration policy instituted several years ago after a contaminated batch entered the United States from its Japanese manufacturer and caused death and illness in a number of individuals. The problem had nothing to do with the tryptophan itself; it had been contaminated by a glitch in its production. In the health food store you can obtain 5-hydroxy-tryptophan, which is a metabolic equivalent; your evening dose of it would be 50 milligrams.

The research that validated the use of tryptophan for sleep was carried out by Dr. Richard Wurtman and his group at the Massachusetts Institute of Technology.[2] The same work also produced the finding that a companion amino acid, tyrosine, is effective in the opposite way: A certain number of people with depression or various other forms of being down, such as just plain fatigue, were responsive to supplements of tyrosine.

Tyrosine is a companion to tryptophan in the sense that these two amino acids are raw materials from which neurotransmitters are made. Just as tryptophan is the precursor of serotonin, tyrosine is the antecedent of norepinephrine, one of the chief members of the "upper," or stimulant, family of neurotransmitters. Adrenaline (also called epinephrine) is a cousin of norepinephrine; these important message carriers in the body are both synthesized from tyrosine.

The proposition, which seemed unlikely at the time of the initial studies done by Dr. Wurtman and Dr. John Fernstrom,[3] is that the body is somehow incapable of gathering enough tyrosine from its stores in blood and tissues to supply the nervous system with raw material for making norepinephrine. (The body also uses tyrosine to make thyroid hormone, another substance associated with being generally up when there's enough of it and down when there's not.) Given our imagined hierarchy of organs within the body, most researchers thought that if the brain needed tyrosine it would get it from some source within the body's protein pool. It turned out, however, that this is not the case. There are simply no stores readily available for the brain to call upon. The nervous system's need for tyrosine has to be supplied by a daily intake of amino acids containing it. Fernstrom showed clearly that a lack of protein in the morning leads to drastic consequences in the availability of tyrosine for supplying the body's needs during the day. In some individuals this shortage of tyrosine results in depression and lethargy.

If you are depressed or lethargic, you may want to experiment with a tyrosine supplement in the morning. The dose ranges from 500 to 3,000 milligrams. Start with 500 milligrams in the early morning, and every few days increase your dose by 500 milligrams. As long as everything is going smoothly and you don't encounter any negative effects, such as anxiety, you can take as much as 3,000 milligrams. If it works, continue to take the lowest dose at which you achieve a good effect. Needless to say, your tyrosine trial should come after you've tried emphasizing protein at breakfast and lunch with the Circadian Diet.

At health food stores you can get a number of other amino acid supplements, some of which are named to imply that they supply your body with fuel. Since, as we have already discovered, in chapter 4, the idea of burning amino acids (or protein) for fuel is a contradiction in terms, if there are benefits to be had from such supplements, you will best get them by taking them in the morning, when protein has its greatest effect in the body.

Supplements of melatonin, an antioxidant made in the brain at night, can also be used to reinforce circadian rhythm, especially when it comes to sleeping. The measure of melatonin provides one of the best examples of a well-defined circadian rhythm, peaking in the bloodstream between midnight and 3:00 a.m. It has one of the sharpest peaks of all the measurable variations of body chemicals during a twenty-four-hour cycle. During the day the level of melatonin in your bloodstream is quite low, and it remains so until the middle of the night, when it suddenly shoots up, returning to baseline in the morning. Its circadian graph looks like a church steeple. One of the curious aspects of melatonin function in the body is that the slightest exposure to light late at night can knock out this peak.

Taking melatonin has been proposed for many reasons—to restore diminishing levels and forestall aging, to help you sleep, or to restore a circadian rhythm disrupted by jet lag. Some of the arguments presented in *The Superhormone Promise,* by William Regelson and Carol Colman, and in *The Melatonin Miracle* by Walter Pierpaoli, William Regelson, and Carol

Colman, are quite persuasive.[4] Current research points to melatonin as a potentially significant anti-cancer agent as well. Naturally, everyone wants to stay young, sleep well, and not get cancer. Many people with these desires take rather large doses, like 3 milligrams, at bedtime. I think smaller amounts are more reasonable. So you might take ⅓ to ½ milligram to help reset your body's clock when you travel. And if you are looking for potential anti-aging or anti-cancer effects, I'd recommend the same dose taken late in the day.

PRESCRIPTION DRUGS AND CIRCADIAN RHYTHM

Prescription and nonprescription medicines may have an impact on your body clock, and in some cases, their benefits and risks may be altered by the timing of their consumption. How can you tell? The detailed rules of that game are beyond the scope of this book, given that there are literally thousands of prescription medicines in use. Comprehensive medical articles have reviewed the timing of drug administration and its relation to absorption, efficacy, and toxicity as well as the tendency of the drug to act as a timegiver, resetting your clock forward or backward depending on the time of day that you take it.[5] Here are some simple clues:

- If you already know that the drug you are taking has a significant side effect involving sleep, you can bet that it affects circadian rhythm. It may affect serotonin levels, as is the case with certain drugs that influence mood, such as antidepressants.

- Most blood pressure medicines, other than diuretics (water pills), work by influencing a branch of adrenaline chemistry. Stimulant medicines, like those given to children for attention problems, also affect this chemistry. So do asthma medicines, except Cromolyn, and decongestants, which work by influencing the chemistry of adrenaline family neurotransmitters. One of the most potent of these is Theophyllin, which is the stimulant found in tea.

- Steroid medications such as prednisone should be taken in the early part of the day, corresponding to the time when blood levels are normally high.

In no case will you find: "This drug may bother your circadian rhythms" on the label. Still, if you suspect that your medication has circadian effects, it doesn't hurt to ask your physician about the time of day when taking the medicine will produce the most benefit and the least damage.

VITAMIN AND MINERAL SUPPLEMENTS

Vitamins and minerals also affect the efficiency of your day and night chemistry. Many vitamins and minerals are "helper chemicals" that have an enormous impact on how well you process and use your food. They are *essential,* a term that has two meanings here: first, that your body cannot make them and must depend on food as a daily source for them; second, they are extremely important in the fundamental tasks that every healthy animal has to accomplish, including the following:

- Carbohydrate metabolism, or taking apart glucose molecules to recover the sun's energy

- Protein chemistry, in which dietary proteins are completely disassembled and their component amino acids used or reassembled to form all of the materials necessary for growth and complex functioning

- Fat metabolism, where dietary fat is set aside for later use or converted into cell membranes and hormones

- Antioxidant protection, in which we protect our own tissues from being "burnt" by the fire of life and environmental oxidant stressors

In addition to their effects on how you digest and metabolize your food, and therefore on the Circadian Diet, vitamins and minerals play a key role in the prevention of chronic illness. In some instances, they are beneficial in amounts greater than you can obtain from a normal balanced diet. Until a few years ago, the reigning medical theology in the United States was that pills are bad and food is the only proper source of nutrients. But a recent editorial in the *New England Journal of Medicine,* entitled, "Eat Right *and* Take a Multivitamin,"[6] shows that the tide of medical opinion has begun to shift. A growing body of evidence has demonstrated that many vitamins and minerals, when taken in larger doses than are available even in a healthy diet, offer protection against osteoporosis, cardiovascular disease, cancer, and a host of other conditions.

Whether you choose to take supplements is your decision. In the rest of this chapter, I will lay out the key vitamins and minerals I consider important to optimize both the effects of the Circadian Prescription and your health and well-being.

FOLIC ACID AND VITAMIN B-12

In 1969, Dr. Kilmer McCully published a biochemical theory that provided a reasonable explanation for the mechanism by which folic acid, an essential member of the B family of vitamins, alleviates not only birth defects but many other problems, including cardiovascular disease and can-

---

GOING BEYOND THE RDA FOR FOLIC ACID

My aim is to give you simple things you can do to help promote healthy body rhythms. But as we take this trip, I don't want you to miss some of the interesting scenery that goes by. Not knowing about folic acid could be hazardous to your health.

The officially recommended doses of folic acid are less than one-tenth of what I take myself and recommend for my patients. The gap is an example of the difference—sometimes a conflict—between public and private health policy. Historically, public health recommendations for nutrients aim low; they insure levels of intake adequate for preventing outright deficiencies. The national body that sets the Recommended Daily Allowances has only just begun to incorporate into their recommendations the notion that higher doses of certain nutrients can prevent chronic illness.

In addition to the scientific literature about folic acid and chronic illness, what convinces me to shoot high with folic acid intake is that I've repeatedly seen doses in the 10-to-20-milligrams range reverse abnormal pap smears, and I believe that the underlying biology is persuasive with respect to other types of cancers, for which both men and women are at risk. As long as I'm sure of its safety, I am confident in recommending a high dose of folic acid.

cer.[7] In 1976, the first reports by R. W. Smithells and his research group appeared, revealing that folic acid supplementation in pregnant women could prevent serious birth defects.[8] Even back then, these initial findings were solid enough that a reasonable person with a scientific background might have looked at them and thought it likely that they would be confirmed by subsequent studies.

It has now been a number of years since the validation of Smithells's and McCully's work. In the last decade or so, there has been a growing body of research demonstrating folic acid's curative and protective properties in a wide variety of conditions, including cancer, cardiovascular disease, cervical dysplasia, and severe birth defects. Folic acid may also play a role in mood disorders. But the health benefits of folic acid are not yet common knowledge.

I don't buy the argument that if you eat a normal diet you'll get enough. And what's more, no matter how you eat, there are many individuals who cannot achieve the protective effect provided by folic acid unless they take a supplement. (You can read about this in more detail in my book, *Folic Acid: The Vital Nutrient That Fights Birth Defects, Cancer, and Heart Disease,* or on my Web page: http://www.sbakermd.com/info/folic/folic1.htm.)

It's hard to discuss folic acid without talking about vitamin B-12, its partner in a critical function: the conversion of homocysteine, a poisonous by-product of your metabolism, into a helpful nutrient, methionine. The partnership of B-12 and folic acid is the basis for the medical recommendation that people not take large doses of folic acid without at the same time assuring that they have normal vitamin B-12 levels. Folic acid can mask symptoms of vitamin B-12 deficiency, called pernicious anemia in its most severe form. This situation is rare, but there's no point in playing loose with it. Whenever I suggest that patients take large amounts of folic acid, I first make sure their vitamin B-12 levels are normal by measuring their blood level of methylmalonic acid, which is a substance whose transformation in the body requires B-12 as a helper. High levels of methylmalonic acid are a sign of insufficient B-12.

What is a large dose of folic acid? I take 5 milligrams a day, which is more than ten times greater than the Recommended Daily Allowance. In order to get this, you need to buy folic acid in 800-microgram pills—the largest available over-the-counter dose you can find because of the longstanding medical caution based on concern over pernicious anemia—and take six per day.

Besides recommending a large dose of folic acid, I'd also suggest that you take it in the evening. This vitamin is more of a specialist than most of the other essential nutrients, which have multiple jobs on both the day and night shifts. Folic acid, however, acts as if it has a particular franchise as a materials supplier for the nightshift chemistry of repair and regeneration.

ANTIOXIDANTS

You can certainly do the Circadian Diet without nutritional supplements. But if you're like most prudent people these days, you probably take some multinutrient combination of vitamins and minerals. Multinutrient combinations don't exist simply to cover all your bases, although that is one reason for taking them. Advice about supplements tends to move in the direction of multiples because nutrients work together in your chemistry. It's not only reasonable but safer to take all the members of a given team of nutrients together.

Take the antioxidant team. Hundreds of substances from your food help perform the antioxidant task of quenching the sparks from your metabolic fire. Before the availability of pumps and hoses, an old-fashioned fire department would organize a line of people to transport bucket after bucket of water from a tank or pond to the scene of a fire. This bucket brigade is an apt metaphor for your body's system for dealing with oxidative stress, which occurs when oxygen or a host of other greedy environmental agents try to steal electrons from your molecules. When this happens, vitamin C steps forward and gives up its electron instead. Vitamin C then takes one from vitamin E, which reaches for the beta-carotene, the next bucket in the brigade, and so on down the line. Such oxidative damage is the final common pathway for your normal metabolic fire, as well as just about everything harmful that happens in your body, whether it's the aftermath of stubbing your toe, being singed in a flame, or being injured by a virus infection or other inflammatory process.

Just as you need a source of carbohydrates to fuel your fire in the evening, your body can also use a generous supply of antioxidants when that fire is burning. In the summary table at the end of this chapter, I stress the following antioxidant family members for evening use: selenium, vitamin E, vitamin C, beta-carotene, and coenzyme Q10.

MAJOR MINERALS: ZINC, CALCIUM, AND MAGNESIUM

Zinc has been in the news in the last couple of years, thanks to evidence that it may help shorten the duration and intensity of the common cold. This mineral is involved in growth and repair, and it supports immune function. Nevertheless, it's not wise to take large doses of zinc without knowing your zinc status, which can only be measured by laboratory tests. You can safely take a small dose, say 15 to 25 milligrams. Zinc is best absorbed on an empty stomach, which is most likely to prevail in the morning, between meals, or at bedtime.

Calcium is a subject of considerable confusion in modern nutrition and popular science because of the difficulty of assessing two simple questions in a given individual. First, does the person have an overall deficit compared to his or her optimal need? Second, is the calcium that is on board properly distributed in the body's three calcium "compartments"? The compartment of which you are probably aware is the bones, which contain nearly all of your body's calcium. The second compartment is the water of your bloodstream and the spaces between the cells of your body. About one-third of your body's total water content, this fluid forms a kind of ocean in which your body's cells live and are nourished; like ocean water, it is relatively rich in calcium and sodium. (This accounts for the saltiness of blood, sweat, and tears.) The remaining compartment for calcium in your body is the water inside all of your cells, which, like the water inside the cells of all living things, is almost calcium free. So the question of calcium supplementation concerns not only whether there is sufficient calcium in your diet but also whether that calcium is adequately absorbed from your intestine and then properly distributed to bones and tissues without getting into your cells, where it is associated with cell death.

Signs of calcium deficiency may be subtle and occur before the obvious symptoms of weak bones and osteoporosis. Clues to the need for calcium may include irritability and muscle cramps, high blood pressure, an apparent intolerance for magnesium when it is taken as a supplement, breast tenderness in women, and hyperactivity in children.

Magnesium is the shepherd of light. When the sun's energy is captured in green plants, magnesium is there to help guide the energy as it becomes condensed in sugar molecules. When those sugar molecules are disassembled by animals to get the sun's energy back, magnesium is there again as a cofactor in most of the key steps in carbohydrate metabolism, where its partner is vitamin B-6.

The distribution of magnesium in your body's water is the opposite of calcium, so the water inside your body's cells is full of magnesium. Like calcium, the measurement of magnesium in the body is difficult because technical methods for assessing active forms of magnesium inside cells are limited. A variety of symptoms that can be generally described as "being uptight" may indicate a need for magnesium. These includes both the muscular and nervous implications of "uptight": anxiety to the point of panic attacks, insomnia, irritability, hyperactivity, tics, twitches, cramps, constipation, menstrual cramps, difficulty swallowing, and heart palpitations and arrhythmias. Mitral valve prolapse, a common, relatively benign abnormality of heart valve function found most often in slender women, is a magnesium-associated condition that has many of these symptoms, which are responsive to magnesium supplementation.[9]

Because calcium and magnesium supplements tend to be calming and may help you get to sleep, they are best taken in the evening. However, the recommended dietary allowance of up to 1,500 milligrams of elemental calcium for adults amounts to so many pills that you may want to split the dose, taking one-third in the morning and the rest at night.

CHROMIUM AND B VITAMINS

Chromium is an ultra-trace element. Unlike calcium and magnesium, which are relatively abundant in animals, it's present only in tiny amounts. It is this low concentration of chromium rather than its distribution that makes it difficult to measure. When complicated research methods are used to assess chromium status in groups of relatively healthy individuals, it turns out that chromium deficits are quite common. Chromium's most prominent role in human chemistry has to do with the regulation of blood sugar; depending on the individual, chromium supplementation may level out either high or low blood sugar tendencies.

NUTRIENT RECOMMENDATIONS

SUPPLEMENT	ADULT DOSE RANGE	TIME	COMMENT
Folic acid	0.5 to 20 mg	Late evening	Helps nighttime repair. (see text)
Tryptophan	500 to 1,000 mg	Evening	If needed for sleep; take with carbohydrate.
Tyrosine	500 to 3,000 mg	Morning	If needed, for depression or lethargy
Melatonin	0.3 to 0.5 mg	Late evening	For jet lag, sleep or anti-aging.
Calcium	1,000–1,500 mg*	Evening dose greater than morning dose	Calming
Magnesium	200–500 mg**	Evening dose greater than morning dose	Calming
Zinc	15–25 mg	Evening	If needed, best on an empty stomach; may take short term to shorten a cold
Vitamin B-12	2–50 mcg	Evening	Works with folic acid
Vitamin B-1	2–50 mg	With dinner	For carbohydrate metabolism
Chromium	200-600 mcg	With dinner	For carbohydrate metabolism
Vitamin B-2 (riboflavin)	5–50 mg	Split dose evenly, morning and evening	
Vitamin B-3 (niacin)	5–50 mg	Split dose evenly, morning and evening.	
Vitamin B-5 (pantothenic acid)	50–200 mg	Split dose evenly, morning and evening	
Vitamin B-6	5–200 mg	Split dose evenly, morning and evening	

SUPPLEMENT	ADULT DOSE RANGE	TIME	COMMENT
Selenium	200–600 mcg	Evening dose greater than morning dose	
Vitamin E	800 UI	Evening dose greater than morning dose	
Vitamin C	500–10,000 mg	Evening dose greater than morning dose	
Vitamin A	10,000 IU	Morning	
Beta carotene	10,000 IU	Evening dose greater than morning dose	
Coenzyme Q10	60 mg	Evening dose greater than morning dose	

* As the citrate

** As the glycinate, chloride, or citrate

Unless you're allergic to yeast, Brewer's yeast or yeast tablets are a rich source of B vitamins. As I've already explained, yeasts are the masters of carbohydrate chemistry. The study of yeast metabolism was the birthplace of modern biochemistry, including the elucidation of the role of the B vitamins in helping to join and separate molecules in all living things. One difference between yeasts and humans is that yeasts can make their own B vitamins, and we cannot. Another difference is that in a given population one yeast cell is much more likely to be the same as another than is one human being like another. The need for different combinations of B vitamins varies among different people in ways that are not easy to assess by routine blood tests. The idea of providing a safe excess in daily intake has appealed to nutritionally oriented doctors for many years and forms the basis for the recommendations in this chapter.

Because vitamin B-1 and chromium are crucial to the metabolism of carbohydrates, which I hope you'll consume in the evening, I give them a place at dinner in the preceding table. The other B vitamins are so versatile or multipurpose that a fifty-fifty division between morning and evening is fine.

23:00
24:00
25:00
01:00
02:00
03:00
04:00
05:00
06:00
07:00
08:00
09:00
10:00
11:00
12:00
13:00
14:00
15:00
16:00
17:00

WHAT ABOUT OILS?

Supplemental oils include essential fatty acids such as those found in flaxseed oil, primrose oil, cod liver oil, or MaxEPA (fish oil). Although certain complexities in fatty acid chemistry might cause some people to need primrose, borage, or black currant seed oil and many others to require flaxseed oil supplementation, the safest bet for most people is one to three capsules of fish oil per day.

The best time to take supplemental oils is in the morning. At night your liver produces bile, which aids fat absorption. When you start your first morning meal, your gall bladder is filled with bile; it squirts in response to the intake of food. Your gall bladder does its best squirting in the morning, so that is when fat absorption is also best.

Individuals may vary in their needs for specific vitamins and minerals. It may be some time before there are official recommendations about the best time of day to take various supplements, but I'm providing you with some preliminary suggestions.

When you follow the Circadian Diet and boost its effects by keeping your flora healthy and taking a selection of vitamin and mineral supplements, you're already doing a lot to strengthen your circadian rhythm. In the next chapter I outline some simple steps you can take to keep various rhythms in your body in sync with each other.

23:00
24:00
25:00
01:00
02:00
03:00
04:00
05:00
06:00
07:00
08:00
09:00
10:00
11:00
12:00
13:00
14:00
15:00
16:00
17:00
18:00
19:00
20:00
21:00
22:00
23:00
24:00
25:00
01:00

CHAPTER

10

Breathing, Exercise, and Meditation: Achieving Rhythmic Integration

So far I've described two different rhythms related to diet. The first is circadian rhythm, which is directly connected to your need for protein in the daytime and carbohydrates in the evening. The second rhythm, indirectly linked to the phytonutrient contents of certain foods, is the cycle of the seasons. Regardless of the time of year, these phytonutrients contain information that is healthy for your reproductive system.

But life revolves around a multitude of predictable rhythms. All vital bodily functions are rhythmic. They are ultimately anchored in the earth's rhythms, most notably the day and night cycle, the lunar month, the seasons, and the year. I say anchored because the earth's rhythms hold us in an inescapable embrace; our connection to them is fundamental.

When various rhythms in your body are tuned to each other just as your diet is tuned to the day and night cycle, you achieve rhythmic integration. In this state your body is in balance, and you suffer when the rhythms fall out of synchrony. (*Syn* means "together" and "chrony" means "in time," so synchrony means "together in time.") Rhythmic disintegration is poisonous.

RHYTHMIC INTEGRATION AND BALANCE

The connection between two or more rhythms in your body is not simply that they are present in the same person. It has to do with tuning. The proper tuning of your body's rhythms is apparent when they mesh with the perfect timing of a high-performance machine. Think about how important it is that the needle, bobbin, thread, and spindle of a sewing machine move in precise relationship to one another to accomplish even the simplest sewing task. Your body's rhythms should also work together so that time flows through you like cloth through the sewing machine.

FLEXIBILITY AND HARMONY

Modern studies of the heart rhythm itself show us what medical students have known since the invention of the stethoscope: A heart that sounds too much like a machine is in serious trouble. A healthy body is flexible; it constantly fine-tunes its rhythms to achieve harmony. Moment to moment and day to day, these adjustments provide interesting fluctuations that enrich our body's music, just as the sound of a good orchestra is richer than that of a machine. Striving for—but never being locked into—perfect synchrony is the mark of a healthy living system. Staying bound to an invariable rhythm is great for clocks and sewing machines but a bad sign when it comes to your body.

But your body is not a machine; I find it more useful and satisfying to think of it as an orchestra. Your brain waves, your cells dividing, your intestines contracting, your temperature rising and falling, and hundreds of other measurable processes are all parts of this orchestra, and its conductor is your circadian rhythm, tuned daily to the day and night cycle of the earth's rotation. Keep this in mind while we explore the interconnected rhythms of two of the main instruments: your heartbeat (pulse or heart rate) and your breathing.

After diet, breathing is the rhythm over which you have most control. Physicians call a respiratory rate of eighteen breaths per minute normal. But when I talk about rhythmic integration I am not concerned with how respiration relates to the clock. What is important is the relationship between your breathing and your body's other rhythmic activities, such as your heart rate.

Start with an exercise you probably remember from your childhood. Pat your head with one hand and rub your tummy in a circular manner with the other. To make it simple, pat your head once per second. It's likely that you can easily also make sixty circles per minute on your tummy to correspond to the pats on your head. Most people can rub their tummies a bit faster or slower so that the pats and the rubs don't come out exactly even.

Now, try something else. Sit down and slap your right knee with your right hand and just keep repeating it: slap, slap, slap, slap. One, two, three, four; one, two, three, four. Begin slapping your left knee with your left hand at the same rate: one, two, three, four; so both hands are slapping: one, two, three, four.

Okay, that's easy. Now continue the one, two, three, four on your right knee. With your left hand slap your knee on every fourth slap of the right hand. One, two, three, slap both, one, two, three, slap both; one, two, three, slap both; and so on. It's not too hard, is it? It depends on a natural communication between your hands that allows them to work out a harmony in which the relationship of one to the other is fixed in a way that is efficient and pleasing.

Take it one step further. Continue the one, two, three, four on your right knee. At the same time, try doing just one, two, three, evenly spaced, on your left side; that is, three slaps on the left for every four on the right. Can't do it, can you? When the relationship between the two hands slapping isn't an even beat, it's too difficult for most people to do, except for trained percussionists, because just about everybody is naturally locked into synchrony.

There is some flexibility. What you were doing with patting your head sixty times a minute and rubbing your tummy a bit faster or slower was asynchronous. You can also choose to live out of sync with the day and night cycle, for example by staying up and eating late at night and sleeping during the day or by working a rotating shift. Being flexible is often convenient and sometimes necessary.

The flip side of that flexibility is that given the chance and the proper timegivers—light, food, and activity—your body will always tend toward harmony. Remember, your internal clock has an approximately twenty-four-hour day that is reset every day to stay in sync with the planet. You can choose to be in or out of harmony, but you can't make disharmony work for you, just as you can slap your knees at different tempos, but you can't make it sound right. The timing on your knees could be one to four, two to four, four to four, or eight to four, but the key is that when you divide the beat on one knee by the beat on the other, you get an even result. If dividing the two rates gives you an uneven answer, the asynchronous tempo will sound wrong.

Human beings have a good ear for that sound. We use it to tune up motors, tune instruments, listen to music, and keep an ear on anything that repeats itself to see if it is properly adjusted. It's hard to argue that something that is out of sync is preferable because as a general rule of nature, things that are in sync sound and work better.

RHYTHMIC INTEGRATION AND FITNESS

It's clear what this has to do with music and machines, but what is its relevance to your body? Assume that your right hand corresponds to the beat of your pulse (your heart rate). Your pulse is one of three measurements that doctors call vital signs. The others are respiration and temperature. It's interesting that they each have a discrete circadian rhythm, but what's more important is that pulse and respiration have a distinctive rhythmic integration.

Go ahead and slap your right knee at a normal pulse rate of, just to make it simple, sixty beats per minute. Now assume that your left hand slapping your left knee is your breathing rate. To be fair, let's not do this when you are talking or doing something else where you might be holding your breath or breathing irregularly. Instead, we'll count your breathing when you are sleeping, resting quietly, out taking a nice walk at a regular pace, or engaged in rhythmic exercise.

Who do you think will fare better, the person who has pulse and breathing tuned so that they work together and are in harmony or the person whose rhythms are all over the place so they are not well synchronized? Common sense and experience with walking, running, music, and other rhythms tells you that a system in harmony performs better than one that isn't.

Besides, researchers have shown that rhythmic integration is connected to better fitness. Dr. Gunther Hildebrandt did an experiment where he studied rhythmic harmony and physical fitness.[1] He asked 140 people to do a brief, standardized workout (the Step Test). Then, over a span of time, including periods of rest and sleep, he measured their pulse and respiration rates. He averaged the measurements and divided pulse rate by respiration rate to obtain their ratio.

Dr. Hildebrandt found that in some people the pulse rate divided by respirations, for example, 60 divided by 15, came out to a whole number such as 4, 5, or 6. In others, the ratio wasn't even. Instead of a whole number such as 4 it resulted in a fraction, like 4.7 or 3.9. The two rates were not in synchrony; if they had been transformed into sounds, they wouldn't have sounded right.

Next he studied two groups of people to see whether they were in comparable shape. The measure he used was how quickly they recovered from the Step Test. If someone's pulse didn't go up much during the activity and quickly returned to its resting state, it demonstrated that he or she was in good shape. On the other hand, when someone's pulse rate shot up during the activity and then took a long time to come down, it was a sign that he or she was in worse condition.

The results were striking. People who had whole number ratios were consistently in better condition. Dr. Hildebrandt's conclusion was that a state of harmony between the rhythms of pulse and respiration is associated with a higher degree of fitness. You can also put it the other way around. If you are in good shape, you are more likely to have harmony between these two vital signs. And while vital signs are already of great interest to doctors, in the next few years it's likely that vital rhythms and synchrony will be of even more interest because harmony is healthier than disharmony.

Please don't leap to the idea that I'm going to ask you to walk around consciously counting your breaths and measuring your pulse until you can make it all come out even. Of course, you do exercise some control over your respiration, since you can consciously choose to hold your breath, breathe fast or slow, regularly or irregularly. But what I want you to do is precisely the opposite: relinquish control over your breathing as a way of achieving rhythmic integration. If you simply relax your breathing, your body will take care of the rest.

BREATHING WITH YOUR DIAPHRAGM TO
ACHIEVE RHYTHMIC INTEGRATION

There are two ways to breathe, although most people know only one. Try this: Take a deep breath by taking air into your lungs so that your chest rises and your shoulders go up. When I ask patients sitting on my examining table to take a deep breath, this is almost invariably what they do.

After you have done this a few times, try breathing with your diaphragm. If you have studied yoga, are a singer, or play a wind instrument, you know how to breathe with your diaphragm. But many of us neglect this important muscle lying between the chest and the abdomen; it is often denied any opportunity to work because the chest muscles are taking care of breathing.

Although it is a muscle, the diaphragm doesn't look like one. It's more like a dome or the top of a balloon, made out of muscle instead of rubber. Your esophagus passes through the diaphragm to deliver food to your stomach. The diaphragm forms a complete barrier between your lungs above and your abdominal cavity below. Its edges are connected around your ribs in the front and back of your body. When the diaphragm muscle contracts, its dome flattens and descends, pushing down on your abdominal organs and pulling down on your lungs, which then expand with air. When you exhale, the dome of the diaphragm relaxes and rises.

Here's how to let your diaphragm do your breathing for you. It's important to become conscious of its efforts and to encourage them, while making sure that your chest muscles don't interfere. Lie down on the floor on your back. Relax and breathe quietly. Place your hand on your abdomen, and take a deep breath; you should feel your hand rise. If you find your abdomen falling when you inhale, then you are breathing in your chest and have a way to go to get the knack of diaphragmatic breathing. When you correctly contract your diaphragm, it pushes your stomach and intestines downward, and there is no place for them to go but out. If you place your other hand on your chest it should stay absolutely still. Take another a deep breath so that your chest barely moves but your abdomen expands in order to accommodate the descent of your diaphragm. Don't stick your abdomen out, just let your diaphragm come down and push it out from the inside.

If you haven't tried this before, you may be surprised to find that it doesn't come naturally; this is because you are so used to breathing with your chest muscles that your diaphragm has nearly forgotten how to do its job. Many of us don't breathe diaphragmatically because going around with your stomach sticking out is considered unattractive. But to breathe properly, getting good deep breaths using your diaphragm, you do need to relax your abdominal muscles.

Once you've learned to relax your breathing and let your diaphragm do the work, you will gain a number of benefits. The diaphragm has a nerve that runs straight up to your brain, where it ends in a place that makes communication between the timing of your diaphragm and your heart possible on an entirely subconscious basis. As long as you don't tell your brain otherwise—by holding your breath or breathing with your chest—your diaphragm will make use of its nerve connections and settle down to a restful pace that is automatically coordinated with your heartbeat at a ratio very close to a whole number. You will be encouraging your body into a state of rhythmic harmony and at the same time promoting the normal release of carbon dioxide from your body, increasing the efficiency of all bodily functions, and improving your performance, especially when you are under stress. And, as you've already seen, the extent to which these rhythms are integrated is directly related to your fitness.

DIAPHRAGMATIC BREATHING, CIRCADIAN RHYTHMS, AND EXERCISE

Breathing properly is especially important when it comes to any performance involving timing and coordination, including exercise. There's a great deal of evidence showing that regular exercise strengthens immunity, controls weight, and lowers the risk of serious illnesses, like cardiovascular disease, diabetes, osteoporosis, and some cancers. It also relieves mild depression and promotes a sense of well-being. What's not so well known is that the way you breathe has an effect on your athletic capacity. Athletes who have been trained to breathe diaphragmatically in training and competition have increased their performance by as much as 10 percent.[2]

You can also apply some rules derived from research on circadian rhythms to get more out of your exercise. The first rule is that the time of

23:00
24:00
25:00
01:00
02:00
03:00
04:00
05:00
06:00
07:00
08:00
09:00
10:00
11:00
12:00
13:00
14:00
15:00
16:00
17:00
18:00
19:00
20:00
21:00
22:00
23:00
24:00
25:00
01:00
02:00
03:00
04:00
05:00
06:00
07:00
08:00
09:00
10:00
11:00
12:00

CIRCADIAN RHYTHMS AND MONDAY NIGHT FOOTBALL

Research on strength, flexibility, reaction time, and aerobic capacity suggest that athletic performance peaks in the late afternoon. A study reported in 1997 in the journal *Sleep* examined whether circadian rhythm could provide a meaningful advantage in competitive athletic events.[3]

The researchers looked retrospectively at twenty-five years of National Football League Monday night football games. They hypothesized that West Coast teams would have an advantage over East Coast teams, regardless of whether the games were played on the east or west coast or the direction either team had to travel. At the time, games began at 9:00 p.m. Eastern Standard Time. Since there is a three-hour time difference between the East Coast and the West Coast, this meant that by their circadian clocks, the West Coast teams were starting the games at 6:00 p.m., close to the theoretical peak of human athletic performance. On the other hand, East Coast teams began playing at 9:00 p.m. on their body's clock and often played until midnight, which is close to the lowest point of human athletic performance.

The results? West coast teams won more often and by more points per game than East coast teams; they also performed significantly better than the predicted Las Vegas point spread for each game. The researchers' analysis ruled out other possible explanations, including the teams' past and present records, injuries, home field advantage, playing surface, jet lag, and travel. The study shows very nicely that picking the right time of day to synchronize your activity with its circadian optimum can make a big difference in the outcome.

day when most people enjoy maximum muscle strength and aerobic capacity—and therefore their best potential for physical performance—is between midafternoon and early evening, so exercise right after work, if possible.[4] And exercise is a timegiver, so you should avoid being out on the tennis court at 11 p.m. just because that is when you can get a court.

The second rule may seem to contradict the first, but it applies mostly to competitive athletes: Be sure to practice at the same time of day that you intend to perform, or as close to that time as possible. The notion underlying this idea is entrainment; it is fundamental to circadian rhythm.[5] Entrainment gives human beings a powerful mechanism to overcome built-in circadian rhythms. You can deliberately establish a pattern that will strengthen your performance at a given time if you regularly train at that time.

Entrainment allows performers and athletes to accomplish a lot. Still, it is not powerful enough to completely sidestep circadian rhythm. For example, entrainment could not overcome the built-in performance deficit that would occur if you tried to compete athletically in the middle of the night when your body is supposed to be doing restoration and repair. And once you've exercised the power of entrainment and established a particular time of day for high performance, it becomes somewhat automatic; to change it again requires further efforts.

MEDITATION AND RHYTHMIC INTEGRATION

It would be gratifying if there were instruments that enabled you to hear how well your body was tuned. But it's even better that you can trust nature to come through with the right harmony if you withdraw interference. That's why sleeping helps restore harmony; you withdraw speech or other conscious efforts and stop breathing with your chest, all of which may interfere with the natural integration of your body rhythms. Rhythmic exercise, done properly and with good diaphragmatic breathing, also encourages rhythmic integration. Another powerful tool for achieving rhythmic integration is meditation.

To get the knack of meditation, find yourself a private corner away from traffic or at least trafficked only by people who won't laugh at you or bother you with questions. Sit in a comfortable chair, but don't lie down; that will tell your body that you are going to sleep, which is a strong possibility when you are learning to meditate. Make sure that both feet are on the floor, and allow your hands to fall together naturally on your lap.

Now, take an inventory of all the muscles in your body, starting with your toes; you wiggle them with the idea of having them nicely relaxed when you are done wiggling. Do the same thing with your arches, ankles, calves, knees, thighs, hips, and pelvis. Pay particular attention to the muscles of your lower pelvis, the ones you usually use for bodily functions; make sure that there is no tension left in them beyond what is necessary to maintain your dignity. Work your way up your body by tensing and relaxing your abdominal muscles, taking a deep breath and making sure that you are breathing with your diaphragm. Get your shoulders, arms, hands, fingers, and neck relaxed. Don't forget to relax your face, since most of us spend some amount of muscular effort every day maintaining an intelligent expression.

Now that you have relaxed as many muscles as you can, working up from your toes to your scalp, you are ready to use your brain in a way that has been available to you all your life but that you have not yet discovered. It's as simple as getting your car into reverse, although reverse is not an apt description, because you are actually going to be moving ahead by learning this new and simple skill, which I think everyone should learn in grade school, along with subtraction and addition. The trick is to enter a meditative state by having your brain set aside three of the activities that usually take up most of its resources. Not only will you find this extraordinarily refreshing, you will allow your body to resynchronize some of the rhythms that might have gotten out of harmony in the harried exercise of your daily routines.

Once you are sitting in a restful position with your muscles relaxed, you have already set aside one of the brain's activities, which is maintaining an intelligent expression on your face or some posture of your body that is bent to a particular purpose. There are only two things left that you need to do or, to put it better, to undo. About 90 percent of your brain's resources are spent on making a three-dimensional color picture of the world around you. It's an extraordinary feat if you think about it, one which you don't ordinarily suspend during waking hours. By closing your eyes, you will quiet your brain's expenditure of energy on three-dimensional color vision. Bingo, you have suspended two of the brain's main chores—muscular activities and vision.

The third step may take a little practice. The problem is that voice inside your head. Now, I don't mean that in a bad way. Everyone has this voice; we call it thinking. In fact, for most of us, it is an extremely unpleasant event if the voice stops talking. If you have ever experienced a blank mind you know that it is terrifying and that sometimes extreme measures such as banging your head on the wall are required to get something going that is better than having nothing at all. Most of us, most of the time, are in control of this voice, although we do sometimes let our thoughts wander and inappropriate thoughts do occasionally occur, like when you get the giggles during a lecture or religious service where dignity, or at least silence, is expected.

It is not feasible for you to simply sit there and stop thinking. Whatever you stop thinking about will be replaced by something else. If you stop contemplating what you forgot to pick up at the dry cleaner you will probably start considering tomorrow's meeting at work or what's for dinner tonight. What you need is a way to keep the language center of your brain busy without letting it actually engage in thinking. The trick is to say a word over and over without allowing your brain to attach meaning to the word because that will engage a train of associations and start you thinking all over again. You can make up a word if you want, but anything you make up will probably have some unconscious meaning that will get you hooked into a train of thought sooner or later. Many people choose the all-purpose word that's constituted by the sound of the letter "M." This is the first sound that babies make when they are learning to articulate. Its early appearance in our vocabulary probably has something to do with the fact that it runs deep into our consciousness and grabs our language centers in a way that other sounds may not.

So, sit with your eyes closed in a completely relaxed, neutral posture and say the letter "MMMMMMMMMM." If you prefer, you can put a letter *O* in front of it, making the sound "OM." You don't need to say it out loud; just say it to yourself. But continue to say it, keeping the language gear of your brain busy. Eventually, this technique will help you keep your mind clear. At first, thoughts will break through. This is perfectly natural so don't fight them, just let them slide past and go back to your "M." As you continue to practice, it will become easier to let the thoughts go, and you will enter a state of consciousness unlike anything else you've ever experienced, a calm, relaxed, waking state that I believe is the hallmark of synchronized body rhythms. Once you are used to doing this meditative exercise, you may even sense the moment when your body becomes resynchronized. At the very least, when you get up to go about your business your refreshed state won't surprise you if you understand what you've just done.

Circadian rhythm is one of many natural cycles that affect your health. When you integrate your circadian rhythms you achieve a harmony that is like good music. If you were able to translate your most important body rhythms into musical tones and chords, you'd be able to hear the tuning of your body as if you were listening to a guitar, of which one earful is enough to tell you whether the tuning is right or wrong.

In the future I believe there will be ways in which you can have your body tuned when your rhythms are asynchronous. But right now you can tune yourself and encourage rhythmic integration in your body by following the Circadian Prescription.

24:00
25:00
01:00
02:00
03:00
04:00
05:00
06:00
07:00
08:00
09:00
10:00
11:00
12:00
13:00
14:00
15:00
16:00
17:00
18:00
19:00
20:00
21:00
22:00
23:00
24:00
25:00
01:00

CHAPTER

11

Losing Weight with the Circadian Diet

The primary reason for going on the Circadian Diet is to improve your short- and long-term health, vitality, and well-being. However, losing weight is a desirable and nearly effortless bonus for many people. This is not an insignificant benefit, since more than one-half of all Americans aged 20 to 74 are overweight, and one-fifth are obese.[1]

Overweight is defined as weighing 10 to 20 percent more than desirable body weight; anything over that is considered obese.[2] Here's a simple formula you can use to see if you're overweight.

For men:

1. Starting point: 106 pounds.

2. Add 6 pounds per inch for every inch of your height over 5 feet (60 inches). This will give your ideal body weight.

3. Take 10 percent of your ideal body weight and add it to the amount in step 2. Anything above this total is overweight.

Take, for example, a man who is 5'10" (70 inches) tall:

Starting point:	106 pounds
Add 6 pounds x 10:	60 pounds
Ideal body weight:	166 pounds

10 percent of ideal body weight: 16.6 pounds

Threshold for being overweight: 182.6 pounds

The formula for women is different:

1. Starting point: 100 pounds.

2. Add 5 pounds for every inch over five feet. This will give your ideal body weight.

3. Take 10 percent of ideal body weight and add it to the amount in step 2. Anything above this total is overweight.

On the Circadian Diet you can shed pounds gradually; at very little emotional cost, you will gain the immense rewards in health and well-being that weight loss can bring. Those benefits are particularly important if you have what are called comorbid conditions. Being overweight is considered a "morbid," or sickly, condition, and comorbid conditions affect 72 percent of people who are 20 percent over their ideal body weight. These comorbid conditions include diabetes, high blood pressure, elevated cholesterol and trigylcerides, coronary artery disease, gallstones, respiratory and sleep problems, degenerative joint disease (arthritis), and certain forms of cancer, including breast, colon, rectal, cervical, endometrial, gallbladder, ovarian, and prostate. Quite a list. In fact, obesity-related conditions, which are responsible for approximately three hundred thousand deaths each year, are second only to smoking as a preventable cause of death.

Even a relatively small amount of weight loss can help a great deal. In one study, for example, "weight loss of any amount" was associated with a 20 percent reduction in all causes of death, a 40 to 50 percent reduction in death from obesity-related cancers, and a 30 to 40 percent reduction in death from diabetes-associated problems. Generally, though, obesity experts—such as Robert H. Lerman, M.D., Ph.D., formerly associate clinical professor of medicine at the Boston University School of Medicine and now research associate at HealthComm International, whose work informs this chapter—recommend setting weight loss goals of 10 to 20 percent of your weight.[3]

THE SIMPLE EQUATION FOR LOSING WEIGHT

There's no magic to losing weight. It hinges on a simple equation—you've got to take in fewer calories than you expend—and there's no way around it. But the Circadian Diet makes it easier to do this and achieve modest weight loss goals of, say, 10 to 20 pounds. It works by changing the timing of what you eat, allowing you to reduce calories while remaining satisfied and alert in ways that only protein in the morning and at lunch can provide. When you follow this diet, you don't feel hungry or deprived; nor do you suffer the irritability that goes along with self-starvation, something you understand if you're one of the 45 million Americans who go on a diet every year. Eating calorie-dense foods early in the day provides another bonus: During a twenty-four-hour period, the same amount of food taken as a single meal in the morning may be associated with weight loss but when consumed late in the day may cause weight gain.

The Circadian Diet operates slowly and steadily, so it doesn't disrupt your life, and it's easy to follow even when you're on the road or eating meals out. Most important, the Circadian Diet is a long-term approach to eating, so it will help you maintain your weight loss, which is harder to do for most people than losing the pounds in the first place.

Take Ralph Austin, for example, the father of one of my patients. He is an average guy, about 20 percent overweight, who had struggled with various diets in the past. He undertook the Circadian Diet initially not for himself but to provide moral support for his son for whom I'd prescribed the diet. I recommended that they try the Rhythmic Shake for breakfast and a high protein lunch, saving most of their carbohydrates for the evening. Mr. Austin did not restrict all carbohydrates from his breakfast or lunch as he might have done if he were following an all protein and fat diet, to achieve rapid reduction in weight and serum insulin levels. Instead, he simply shifted some of his daytime carbohydrates into the evening. He soon found that he was effortlessly losing weight; he dropped 20 pounds in a couple of months. He reports: "I've lost my hunger. My cravings are ten percent of what they used to be and I haven't been dizzy or shaky; nor do I wake up at night. Sometimes, I forget meal times, which never could have happened before. I keep cheese and nuts available, now that I know what an incredible difference these protein snacks make to me in the mornings."

Mr. Austin is an example of the many overweight people who can accomplish their goals without severely restricting fat or carbohydrates. His story is impressive because he lost weight so quickly. But in the long run, the people who lose weight slowly do the best. When I think of the hundreds of my patients over the last thirty-five years who have, consulting me or others, subjected themselves to various programs for losing weight and maintaining their weight loss, it's evident the gentle therapies work best. People who make a drastic change in their lifestyle, exercise, and eating habits, consult with experts, and join groups for support are more likely to achieve success than those who stay home on the couch and think about it. On the other hand, they don't get the same long-term results as people who make smaller adjustments in eating patterns that keep them feeling comfortable and contented.

With the Circadian Diet, you decide how quickly you want to achieve your weight loss goals. Here are two simple measures that will help you figure it out. First is your caloric expenditure. How much energy do you expend every day by turning food into the fuel for muscular activity, thought, detoxification, and replacing worn-out parts of your body, in other words, living? To find out, if you're a woman, multiply your weight, say 150 pounds, by 11; the result is 1650 calories. If you're a man, use a factor of 12; at 150 pounds, your normal daily caloric expenditure is 1800 calories. Exercise uses up additional calories; these range, for a 150-pound person, from 240 calories per hour for light physical activities such as walking slowly (2 m.p.h.) to 920 calories per hour for running (7 m.p.h.) or other strenuous physical exertion.[4]

Here's the daily caloric expenditure for a woman weighing 150 pounds who does three hours of walking and other light physical activities:

Normal expenditure: 150 pounds x 11   1650 calories

Light physical activities: 240 x 3 hours   720 calories

                        TOTAL   2370 calories expended

Once you've figured your daily caloric expenditure, it's time to look at the other side of the equation, your intake. Use a simple calorie-counting guide to calculate your average daily intake. Keep a detailed record for seven days that includes *everything* you eat and drink. Divide the total by seven to get a rough daily average. If you take in 100 calories per day more than you expend, you will gain approximately 10 pounds in a year. Conversely, if you slide below your energy requirement by a consistent 100 calories per day, you will lose 10 pounds in a year. If you undershoot by 200 calories per day, you lose 10 pounds in six months; and if you take in 400 calories per day less than you require, you will lose 10 pounds in three months. This is the kind of goal that many of us have in mind when we confront the fact that our pants don't fit any more. A loss of 10 pounds translates to about 2 inches off your waist.

"APPLES" AND "PEARS"

Your waist leads me to another twist on the whole issue of obesity. Your appearance may matter a lot to you; it may even be the crucial factor in your decision to take off a few pounds. But the health benefits from weight loss accrue more to people with apple obesity, whose extra pounds are around the waist. Apple obesity is a marker for insulin resistance and its attendant health woes, as well as other comorbid conditions.

Pear obesity, in which the main distribution of weight is in your buttocks and thighs, is relatively free of health risks, as long as your waist measurement is less than 39 inches. Pear obesity may be distressing if you are a woman plagued by the fashionable emphasis on slender hips and thighs in females. And you will certainly feel better if you shed some extra weight, no matter where it is. But you are in a different category from, say, the men with big beer bellies, whose weight gain is mostly inside the abdominal wall in the form of a grossly fat omentum. The omentum is an apron of tissue that hangs across the upper part of the abdomen in front of the intestines, forming a kind of greasy padding between the inside of the abdominal wall and the underlying coils of the intestines. Its normal function is to provide some protection when the intestines are perforated by disease or piercing wounds from the outside. It is one of the preferred places for deposits of the kind of unwanted fat that is associated with diseases of carbohydrate metabolism, like insulin resistance and the comorbid conditions mentioned earlier.

INSULIN RESISTANCE AND WEIGHT GAIN

Insulin resistance is also one of the genetic factors connected with obesity. Some people who are overweight have more trouble achieving and maintaining their weight loss goals than others. Often, this is because genetic traits are in a tug-of-war with exercise and diet when it comes to determining how big your body will be. If you look at your family and conclude that you are the victim of genetic destiny because many of your relatives are obese, then you may indeed have a harder time reaching your statistically ideal body weight. Your chances of success will be better, however, if you focus on the one factor likely to be predisposing you and your family to obesity—insulin resistance, the tendency to bump up your serum insulin whenever carbohydrates become available.

As pointed out in chapter 4, your ancestors' ability to increase their serum insulin levels was an advantage in days when food supplies were short and starchy carbohydrates were scarce. Today, when carbohydrates are considered staples of the diet, and a particularly heinous form of carbohydrates—junk foods—are the staple of many people's diets, this ancient survival trait has turned against you.

Whether your insulin resistance is connected to apple obesity, genetics, or both, your best bet is the Circadian Diet. Not only will it help you lose weight, it will also reduce your risk of developing the health problems associated with this disorder. As I've already mentioned, the diet brings down your serum insulin levels by less frequent ingestion of carbohydrates. So move carbohydrates out of your daytime meals as much as possible, and move most of your protein to breakfast and lunch. And to lose weight, keep your daily calorie intake at least 100 calories below your energy requirements.

From a public health point of view, the problem of obesity is simple. In the last fifteen years the average weight of American adults has increased by about 8 pounds,[5] thanks to too little exercise and diets too high in fat and carbohydrates. If everyone who went on a diet successfully lost those 8 or more pounds, the gains in health and the savings in the cost of obesity-associated illness would be enormous. The ironic thing is that it seems that everyone is on a diet. It's likely that you're one of those people and that you've lost the 8 pounds, possibly more than once, but that you keep gaining them back because you do not make a permanent change in your eating habits.

When desperation leads to diets that are extreme in their restriction of calories, protein, or carbohydrate, it can spell either trouble or failure. The Circadian Diet is a recipe for moderation; my experience with it suggests that it is the approach most compatible with success in both the short term and the long run. Eating protein in the morning promotes biochemical and hormonal changes that make it possible to lose weight and remain satisfied. And because it's easy to do and they feel better, most of my patients stick with the diet over the long haul.

24:00
25:00
01:00
02:00
03:00
04:00
05:00
06:00
07:00
08:00
09:00
10:00
11:00
12:00
13:00
14:00
15:00
16:00
17:00
18:00
19:00
20:00
21:00
22:00
23:00
24:00
25:00
01:00

CHAPTER

12

Women

More than men, women's lives are defined by divisions of time. These divisions include events marking the beginning of reproductive life, the three seasons that represent the length of a pregnancy, and the years before and after children gain independence, all of which may vary considerably from one woman to another. The timing that binds all women together is the monthly cycle. Recent findings showing that components of certain foods in the diet, like isoflavones and lignans, have an impact on the hormones that regulate the menstrual cycle and offer women another option besides taking hormones for maintaining control over their own bodies.[1]

Hope Wheeler is a fifty-year-old middle school teacher and counselor, a sweet, even-tempered, intelligent woman. I first treated her several years ago for Crohn's disease, in which the small intestine and its associated lymph nodes become chronically inflamed and provoke symptoms of pain and diarrhea. Hope had already seen another doctor, but she didn't want to take the many drugs that had been prescribed. Working together, we changed her diet, and within weeks we saw positive results. These days, she may occasionally have a bout of her illness, but she is much better.

Recently Hope began to have symptoms of menopause. Her gynecologist put her on hormone replacement therapy (HRT) because she was having hot flashes, headaches, and difficulty concentrating; she also was not sleeping well. When I saw her, she was concerned because she had stopped getting her period. (When a woman takes both estrogen and progesterone, which is the preferred hormone therapy for menopause, she may still expect to bleed every month.)

I recommended that Hope drink the Rhythmic Shake for breakfast. Although she was skeptical, our successful history treating her Crohn's disease encouraged her to try what seemed like an unlikely solution. The following month her period returned, and she has been menstruating ever since. And Hope was pleasantly surprised to find that she had more energy and no longer felt drained at midmorning.

As an adjunct to her HRT, Hope is now following the other rules of the Circadian Diet, eating a high protein lunch and saving carbohydrates for evening. And she has started giving her ten-year-old daughter the shake, getting her off to a good start every morning, too.

It's not that all women's health issues are defined by monthly periods. But the question of periods themselves—their regularity, frequency, duration, and obvious connection to successful fertility—does apply specifically and only to women. And it's hard to imagine any improvement or decline in the health of a young-adult-to-middle-aged woman that doesn't have some bearing on her reproductive system and its cycles. Constipation, bloating, breast tenderness, breast lumps, irritability, vaginal yeast infections, fatigue, depression, changes in libido, cold hands and feet or feeling cold all over, allergies, changes in body weight, and fluid retention all are common symptoms for which women regularly report cyclic changes.

Like Hope Wheeler, many of my female patients have successfully used the Circadian Diet to free themselves from a variety of these symptoms. And many of the larger issues—breast, uterine, and ovarian cancers, infertility, menopause, pregnancy, and weight control—also have rhythmic aspects that make them responsive to the diet's effects.

PREMENSTRUAL SYNDROME (PMS)

The circadian (daily) connection to menstrual (monthly) periods embraces one of the fundamental considerations in this book: All your numerous body rhythms are interconnected, so if you strengthen one rhythm you tend to positively affect the others. Just as a strong drummer in a band will sway the other musicians' tempos, a strong circadian rhythm will have a positive influence on other body rhythms, even those that, like the twenty-eight-day menstrual cycle, have quite a different frequency. To argue the contrary defies common sense as well as research on rhythmic integration, which I discussed in chapter 10. When I treat a woman with premenstrual syndrome, irregular periods, or infertility, I translate her complaint into "I've got a broken rhythm." And I try to help her fix it by working to repair all the rhythms I can.

A few years ago, common thinking was that premenstrual syndrome (PMS) was all in women's heads. (Attention deficit disorder in children is a similar story.) Then the struggle to have it recognized as a legitimate diagnosis turned it into a singular "entity" rather than a collection of symptoms resulting from being in some way out of balance. The balance question is especially troublesome for women who are frequently told that their problem derives from a "hormonal imbalance" that can be treated by taking hormones in the form of birth control pills. But this remedy may successfully hide the problem as well as the real cause.

Unfortunately, a search for the real cause is fruitless if you're looking for the same cause in different women. The normal rise of progesterone that precedes periods does not necessarily go unnoticed by any woman who is sensitive to changes in her body. But the changes in body chemistry that cause discomfort, distress, and a wide variety of other symptoms may be driven by all sorts of problems, from food allergies to special needs for magnesium.

Given the carbohydrate craving that frequently accompanies PMS, it's not surprising that the answer for many women lies in the hormonal consequences of achieving dietary balance. This means making sure that you get those things for which your body may have special needs and avoiding the things that are bothersome for you. And for several reasons, the Circadian Diet really shines brightly when it comes to menstrual problems. By emphasizing protein in the morning and saving moderate carbohydrate consumption for the evening, you will reinforce your day and night rhythm, which will in turn strengthen your monthly cycle. In addition, the omega-3 oils in the diet favor your prostaglandin hormone chemistry, while the soy protein and flaxseed fiber modulate your steroid hormone chemistry.

Many women need do no more to achieve good results than simply follow the diet. Beyond that, the remedy for PMS that works most often is generous supplements of vitamin B-6 and magnesium, which are two of the key nutrients involved in body chemistry in general and, for reasons that are not completely understood, have a special effectiveness against the symptoms of tension and irritability that characterize PMS. I recommend adding to your daily regimen 50 milligrams of vitamin B-6 in the form of pyridoxal phosphate and magnesium in doses ranging from 200 to 600 milligrams per day of elemental magnesium, depending on the form of magnesium you take.

MENSTRUAL IRREGULARITY AND THE CIRCADIAN PRESCRIPTION

Because reinforcing a strong circadian rhythm sways other rhythms of your body toward constancy and stability, the Circadian Prescription helps menstrual irregularity. And the flaxseed and soy protein in the diet magnify the benefit. For example, studies have shown that women taking flaxseed supplements had an overall decrease in ovarian dysfunction and that they ovulated more regularly, which in turn lowered their risk for breast cancer.[2]

It's also important to focus on other general principles of rhythmic living when trying to remedy menstrual irregularity. Eating, sleeping, waking, and exercise are the activities over which you have the most control. The Circadian Diet takes care of eating. Other rhythms to strengthen include regular times for going to bed and awakening, daily bowel movements, rhythmic exercise, especially in the afternoon, and daily exposure to the outdoors. Full spectrum sunlight is the strongest influence on your circadian rhythm, so expose yourself for one-half hour a day, close to dawn or dusk. There are no commercially available lenses that transmit the full spectrum of natural light, so you should do this with minimal use of glasses. Finally, I'd suggest Tai Chi or other exercises designed to promote normalization of body energy, as well as meditation and exercising to music. All of these steps will go a long way toward reinforcing a strong body rhythm, which will then nudge your other rhythms toward regularity.

FERTILITY

As part of the Circadian Prescription, the measures just described can also be used to treat infertility. While the treatment of infertility has become an extraordinarily high-tech, expensive, and emotionally exhausting experience for many women, I believe that one of the reasons for the relatively high incidence of infertility is our general departure in modern life from the rhythmic patterns so evident in the lives of people who live in traditional societies. No one who has lived in a remote village where everything is done by hand can fail to notice how most of the people's activities are rhythmic. Living in the 1950s in the valley of Katmandu, Nepal, where neither machines nor animals were available for farming, and later, while serving in the Peace Corps in Africa, I witnessed the daily round of walking, tilling, planting, weeding, threshing, milling, grinding, beating, singing, chanting, and praying. Each activity took place at its regular time between sun-up and sundown, depending on the season.

During my two years providing prenatal care and outpatient gynecology in Africa, I saw well-nourished women living in an agricultural milieu who sometimes had problems with fertility because of infectious disease. But it was rare to find a woman who couldn't conceive if "all the tests" were normal. This is not the case in women I see in this country, where the notion of "all the tests" includes gynecological measures but ignores the potential influence of diet on hormone balance.

If you are concerned about fertility, you should certainly pay attention to your rhythmic and hormonal balance. Many infertile couples have problems resulting from rather subtle changes in their hormonal chemistry of the vague type referred to as "hormone imbalance," mentioned earlier. This being the case, and the relationships among diet, intestinal flora, hormones, and cellular physiology being what they are, adjusting these factors is the place to begin. Of course, you should also have a basic infertility workup to ascertain that anatomical considerations, such as blocked Fallopian tubes or inadequate egg production or sperm counts are not the problem. And considering the importance of the prostate in providing a medium in which sperm do their work, men in infertile couples should pay attention to the issues discussed in chapter 14.

But most of all, given the impact of yeast and other abnormal intestinal germs on hormonal balance, I encourage you to make a serious effort to clear up any problems of this type before preceding further. When I first encountered infertile couples who made babies after clearing up an intestinal or vaginal yeast problem I thought that it worked simply because of a general improvement in the woman's health and nutrition. More recently, however, the research on the relationship between robust intestinal flora and healthy hormones has helped me understand that controlling yeast and normalizing intestinal germs may be a highly specific remedy for the infertile woman.[3]

Sometimes this seems laughably easy. It's always problematic when doctors give curbside advice, but when the curb was between me and my neighbors Betty and Leo, I couldn't resist my instinct to be helpful when the question of their infertility came up. They had already gone through a complicated workup and treatment plan that had failed to bring results. Meanwhile, Betty had been chronically troubled by horrendous hives. Based on a brief history, I thought there might be a connection between her rash and the infertility. Indeed, Betty's hives responded dramatically to a yeast-free diet and antifungal medicine, and she soon became pregnant.

POLYCYSTIC OVARIES

Besides PMS, menstrual irregularity, and infertility, hormone imbalance is connected to polycystic ovaries and the associated symptoms. Often, women with this troublesome condition get answers from their doctors along these lines: "You have a hormone imbalance, but your tests are not all *that* abnormal."

It's true that many forms of hormonal expression—differences in skin texture and breast size as well as menstrual regularity or irregularity, for example—simply do not show up in hormone test results because there is a wide range of "normal." But there are also women whose lab tests lie near the boundary between normal and what a doctor would consider a "condition." These women have distressing symptoms such as apple obesity, acne and oily skin, hirsutism (a tendency for hair to grow where it's not wanted) or baldness, menstrual disturbances, and infertility. They also often experience strong cravings for carbohydrates.

If you fit this description, you may or may not have been told that you have polycystic ovaries. The hormonal imbalance of polycystic ovaries is due in large part to insulin resistance and therefore can be relieved to a significant degree by controlling the amount and timing of your carbohydrates. Polycystic ovaries may leave you feeling that your body—and your life—is out of control, as well as disappointed that all of the hormonal therapies at the disposal of doctors are useless. Given that we usually respect drugs far more than diet, it is a special paradox that the dietary restriction and timing of carbohydrates achieved with the Circadian Diet can have such a strong influence on a condition so resistant to medications.

MENOPAUSE

In North America alone, almost four thousand women become menopausal every day, and 40 million women will pass through menopause during the next two decades.[4] Given that there exists such a clear blood test to determine follicle stimulating hormone (FSH) level to determine the time when menopause begins, many doctors, myself included, have tended to believe that menopause happens all of a sudden. Indeed, periods may stop all of a sudden, lending credence to the myth. But for many women, there is a transitional period—called the perimenopause, from *peri,* meaning "around"—of accumulating symptoms, some of which may not seem at all hormonal.

23:00
24:00
25:00
01:00
02:00
03:00
04:00
05:00
06:00
07:00
08:00
09:00
10:00
11:00
12:00
13:00
14:00
15:00
16:00
17:00
18:00
19:00
20:00

FSH

Follicle stimulating hormone (FSH) is a substance made by your pituitary gland that speaks to your ovaries every month, telling them "make a follicle." The follicle is a puddle of nutrients on the surface of your ovary in which eggs develop while sending back signals to the pituitary gland that the message was received. When eggs and feedback stop arriving, the pituitary starts shouting; thus, FSH levels rise and remain elevated during every woman's postmenopausal career.

Many lab test results have gray zones at their upper or lower limits of normal, and all too often patients with puzzling problems produce gray zone results that detract from the kind of decisiveness that helps a doctor feel confident. Hardly ever do FSH levels fall in a gray zone. They are either low and normal or sky high and menopausal, with no overlap among the levels doctors assign to each range.

When Alma Hiatt weaned her last baby at age forty, she developed symptoms that included premenstrual irritability, loss of interest in sex as well as decreased erotic sensitivity, irritable bowel, and headaches. At forty-eight, she came to see me for the increasing severity of her irritable bowel symptoms, which had previously been controlled by antispasmodic drugs prescribed by her gastroenterologist. She was suffering from sleep disturbances and vaginal dryness, and she'd had two or three hot flashes in the month or two before consulting me. But her periods remained steady, and her FSH level was normal.

I checked Alma's FSH level because I feel that dealing with menopausal issues should take top priority in tackling all sorts of health problems in women her age, who might respond to hormone replacement therapy. Indeed, not knowing about someone's menopausal status is an obstacle to caring for any woman who may be approaching menopause. After starting on the Circadian Diet, including the morning shake, Alma's mood, energy, and sleep improved markedly. Although Alma benefited from the dietary changes, including the soy protein and flaxseed, there was still room for improvement. This tipped me off to the notion that her longstanding symptoms, going back to age forty, may have been an expression of perimenopause.

Because the Circadian Diet relieved Alma's hormonal symptoms, I proposed going further with a brief trial of hormone replacement therapy. It was a roaring success; all her other symptoms disappeared. Alma's story provides an example of how problems that appear long before official menopause, including some that may seem unrelated to hormones, such as headaches and irritable bowel, may yield dramatically to the Circadian Diet and other hormonal intervention.

HORMONE REPLACEMENT THERAPY, PHYTONUTRIENTS, AND CANCER

I hear from many women that the notion of menopause and hormonal replacement therapy is fraught with confusion, fear, and indecision. The trouble is that you really do need to make some decisions. So here's an easy one. Decide right now that you will take the flaxseed and soy protein in connection with the Circadian Diet. All health decisions eventually come down to an assessment of the relationship between possible risk and possible benefit. It's easy enough to say that by present reckoning, the benefits of HRT for most women outweigh the risks by a substantial margin. But the benefits—decreased cardiovascular disease and osteoporosis and better cognitive function and memory—somehow don't claim women's attention as much as the high stakes involved in the slightly increased risk of breast cancer.

Until recent research revealed the protective effects of lignans and isoflavones, the risks/benefits/stakes dilemma lacked a middle ground. I still think HRT is a bargain, but when I see the kinds of immediate hormonal benefits, including temporary postponement of menopause as experienced by Hope Wheeler, I am a firm believer that all women can partake in the protection of the Circadian Diet without being spooked by concerns over the stakes. Even if you're undecided about HRT you don't have to hesitate about doing the Circadian Diet.

Phytonutrients will not completely eliminate the risk of breast cancer for all women, since some individuals have a genetic makeup and other risk factors that make a decisive contribution. However, the present weight of evidence that we all must use to make choices today about our future health makes it look far safer to include soy protein and flaxseed in our diets than to do nothing. And that's just considering the breast cancer issue. The ingredients in the Circadian Diet regimen are also strongly linked to reduced risk of osteoporosis and cardiovascular disease.

As you know, some of my medical opinions were engendered by my experiences learning and practicing in Africa and the Far East, where my patients' diet, climate, lifestyle, and economics are different from those of the patients I see today. Women living in traditional societies suffer from many disadvantages with regard to personal freedom. But those who eat traditional diets and perform vigorous agricultural and other physical activities go through menopause with far fewer symptoms than women in our society. Of course, these women do sometimes fall into melancholy and ill health for which modern medicine has the remedies. But as a general rule the use of hormone replacement therapy to relieve menopausal symptoms wouldn't have a big market in these cultures.

Because studies have shown that Asian women, whose diets contain significant amounts of soy isoflavones, experience fewer menopausal symp-

THE CIRCADIAN DIET AND REPRODUCTIVE CANCER

The evidence that flaxseed, soy, and other sources of lignans and isoflavones lower the risk for breast and other reproductive cancer has become so convincing that it's hard to choose among all the individual scientific studies that document this connection. You should know, however, that many different kinds of studies have been done, as follows.[5]

- Lower rates of breast cancer have been found in populations whose diets are rich in isoflavones and lignans.

- Lower levels of isoflavones and lignan products have been found in the blood and urine of women with breast cancer than in women without breast cancer, with the implication that their diets contain fewer of these phytonutrients.

- The chemical mechanisms have been discovered by which these phytonutrients restrict the blood supply to cancers, control estrogen excess, and limit the kind of unwanted cell divisions associated with cancerous changes.

- Sixteen animal cancer experiments have shown protective effects of soy, and no studies have shown any negative effects.

- Consumption of soy-rich diets has been shown to reduce blood levels of ovarian and adrenal hormones associated with increased cancer risk, even after as short a period as one month of consumption.

- Studies have shown that genistein, one of the isoflavones found in soy, "may prevent symptoms and diseases associated with estrogen deficiency and . . . inhibit the growth of estrogen sensitive and estrogen independent cancers."

toms, it's no surprise to me that my women patients entering menopause can get symptomatic relief from food-based substances. Thus, while HRT has its place in the long run, the Circadian Diet can provide immediate effects in alleviating the hot flashes, sleep disturbances, fatigue, depression, and difficulty concentrating associated with entrance into menopause.

Sometimes it's hard to know who to ask when making a choice about a treatment. When I see women in such a dilemma, I advise them to ask their own bodies. Whether you're talking about HRT or the Circadian Diet, a one- to three-month trial is an exceedingly low-risk proposition. If during such a trial your own body jumps up and down and says

"Hooray," with the elimination of multiple sources of discomfort and distress, you don't have to ask me whether this is likely to be a good thing for you. The confidence gained by listening to your body can be worth ten expert opinions, newspaper articles, or scary stories from your mother or acquaintances.

23:00
24:00
25:00
01:00
02:00
03:00
04:00
05:00
06:00
07:00
08:00
09:00
10:00
11:00
12:00
13:00
14:00
15:00
16:00
17:00
18:00
19:00
20:00
21:00
22:00
23:00
24:00
25:00
01:00

CHAPTER

13

Children

One of the most creative observations of child development pioneer Arnold Gesell was that the stages of a child's development proceed like a slow dance. A child alternately unfolds into a psychological posture of openness and extension and then closes up again to become more inward and self-protective. The sanity of all parents is enhanced by understanding the timing of these stages of childhood (and adult development as well), in addition to having a firm grasp on circadian rhythms as they apply to your child's sleeping, eating, and behavior.

When I was little I came into regular contact with a lot of grownups because my father was the minister of a church. As one of the minister's two children, I was subject to more attention, praise, criticism, head pats, cheek pinches, lifts into the air, and piggyback rides than most other kids. After a while I realized that most grownups really didn't think that I was very smart. Not that I was stupid, but I was a child, and somehow children, according to the adults, just didn't get it. My favorite grownups were men and women who treated me like someone who could understand what they were talking about and appreciated being accorded the respect due an intelligent life form.

In my adult life I've tried to treat the thousands of children I've known with that kind of respect. This includes children who are nonverbal, both those who are too young to speak and those who for one reason or another are unable to get the knack of language as easily as others. Children are always listening; in fact, their comprehension is often more precise and sensitive than that of adults.

But sometimes, like Billy Malone, children learn best by doing.

Billy is a sandy-haired, broad-shouldered boy with an open face, a direct gaze, a good handshake, and a "glad to see you, Sid" approach when he comes to my office. His breathless enthusiasm propels his speech at a speed that verges on outrunning his thoughts. It might be fun to be with him on a camping trip. But at school they called him a pain in the class. "Hyperactive. Poor attention. Needs Ritalin," they said.

Billy first came to see me a couple of years ago, when he was eight and a half years old, for attention and behavioral issues. He had trouble sitting still, being patient, and thinking clearly. He couldn't talk in a targeted, directed manner or express himself well because he'd go off on tangents.

He'd been taking Ritalin four times a day. But according to his mother, Nora, the effects of the medication, which at first had lasted for four hours, were now wearing off in two. And Billy was experiencing rebound effects; not only did his parents have to medicate him more often, but when the Ritalin wore off he became emotionally labile—teary and sad.

The first clue I seized on when trying to sort out where to begin with Billy was his past history of taking antibiotics. He had been on and off "the pink medicine" for ear aches for most of the first three years of his life, and by the time he was five he had taken seventeen courses of antibiotics. Yeasts, which overgrow in our intestines when we take antibiotics, not only like carbohydrates as their food but make chemicals that interfere with our carbohydrate chemistry. This interference tends to make us crave carbohydrates and be intolerant of them when we have a yeast problem. After Billy responded well to a low yeast diet and a medication to lower the amount of yeast in his intestines, I figured that his remaining daytime inattentiveness could be from poor handling of his breakfast of waffles, fruit, juice, and other high carbohydrate foods. So I suggested he try the shake.

Billy loved the shake at first. But his parents realized that he really needed to chew to feel satisfied and that he missed having something to sink his teeth into. So they sometimes give him smoked salmon, eggs, or tuna fish, and they allow a small amount of carbohydrate with it.

When Billy sticks to the diet, he's much better. Eating protein foods early in the day made a big difference, and the shake has helped even more. He's become much more clearheaded and has improved his performance in school. The dietary changes worked so well that he no longer has to take Ritalin. I believe that a significant number of Ritalin-taking children could become drug free by just loading up on protein at breakfast and saving their carbohydrates for dinner.

THE PIG OUT DIET

Even though Billy felt, behaved, and learned much better immediately after going on the Circadian Diet, during subsequent appointments Billy and Nora acknowledged that he was sliding away from total compliance; he was "getting tired of eating that way." He was still doing pretty well, but Nora was worried that he was getting a little too lax.

Instead of proposing that he tighten up his diet again, which would be the suggestion I'd make to an adult patient, I took advantage of children's fondness for spectacles, such as those afforded by extremes of size or color. Big fireworks, a tiny music box, a huge locomotive, a miniature porcelain horse all fit into children's appreciation of extremes. I recommended that Billy try the Pig Out Diet, which is popular with children and their parents once they understand how it works. It's a refinement of the "let him eat all he wants and we'll see what it does to him" line of action familiar to me from my own childhood. I was subjected to this experiment after annoying my parents by repeatedly suggesting that I had a greater tolerance for potato chips than they thought. Finally, they allowed me to explore the upper limits of my potato chip tolerance. I found it, although I threw up several times along the way, thereby increasing my respect for grownups' understanding of limits and expanding my awareness of the digestive process.

The idea for Billy was to pick a day when school performance and behavior weren't crucial and let him return to his previous eating habits, starting with a large, fairly sweet, high carbohydrate breakfast. Then, he'd be the judge of whether it made a difference.

When Billy tried the Pig Out Diet, he got drunk. Silly, spacey, goofy drunk. Drunk? Yes, in a very real way. The effects of a high carbohydrate load in some children provoke all the kinds of behaviors that you'd find in a tavern where you might encounter happy drunks, sad drunks, hyperactive drunks, silly drunks—all of whom would have difficulty concentrating if they were delivered to a classroom, and each of whom might, at different stages of drinking, pass through different states of intoxication. Many parents with whom I discuss this parallel with their children's difficulties give me a strong flash of recognition. They are more able to understand the connection to carbohydrates and yeast problems when they realize that everything served in the tavern is made from yeast and carbohydrates. The only difference between drinking alcohol and feeding carbohydrates to yeasty children is that the tavern's fermentation is in the brewery and the child's is in his or her digestive tract. Some children are intolerant of carbohydrates without having a yeast problem, and the child's fermentation produces other toxins besides alcohol, but the overall picture is true.

The Pig Out Diet convinced Billy, far more than any word from his mom or a doctor could, that sticking with very low carbohydrate intake in the morning was best for him. I believe that children of any age, even including those under a year, are able to recognize when a change in their diet produces or relieves symptoms. Children over age seven who try the Pig Out Diet are able to take ownership of that observation and acknowledge, however reluctantly, that yes, it does make a difference. For children younger than seven, it's up to the adults to point out that after freely indulging in bagels, donuts, waffles, and juice for breakfast they get a bad case of the "can't-help-its."

THE CIRCADIAN DIET AND THE "CAN'T-HELP-ITS"

The "can't-help-its" is a pediatric diagnosis—often applicable to adults—that came into my repertoire thanks to my close friend Michel Duques, a child therapist. After Michel gave me this wonderful phrase to describe a variety of problems suffered by children, I decided that the "can't-help-its" may be one of the most common problems of contemporary Western civilization. No matter whether it's bedwetting, attention problems, irritability, moodiness, or constipation, the children's cry to grownups is: "I just can't help it." What we'd all really like is a pill for this ailment, so we could take our child to the pediatric neurologist, have the diagnosis confirmed, and receive a simple prescription for a maintenance dose of Help-X.

Kidding aside, one of the toughest issues you face as a parent is deciding when and where to get help for your child. And deciding where to go is crucial because the kind of help you get often shapes the outcome early in the game, sometimes before you even know what your child needs.

Before you seek a specialist's care, I recommend that you try the Circadian Diet, no matter what kind of "can't-help-its" your child has. In my experience, the diet produces positive results in about 50 percent of children, regardless of the problem. I'm talking about children with chronic illness, especially those with symptoms that don't quite add up to a distinctive "diagnosis" but that seem worthy of attention beyond reassurances that he or she will "grow out of it." These include sleep disturbances, problems in bowel function such as constipation and diarrhea, and especially the fluctuations in mood, energy, behavior, attention, and general vitality that often lie in a gray zone where it's hard to decide if there is really something wrong.

ATTENTION DEFICIT DISORDER AND HYPERACTIVITY

The approach I recommend can be beneficial for a broad range of ailments, but I've found it to be particularly successful for children with attention deficit (and hyperactivity) disorder (ADD or ADHD). Attention deficit disorder affects a large group of children who are especially sensitive to something going on in their environment. Whatever these stimuli may be, they probably affect all children, but they affect some more severely than others. The National Institutes of Health estimate that as many as 5 percent of American schoolchildren are affected by ADD;[1] the number is probably significantly higher. In fact, some experts suggest it is as high as 10 percent.[2]

The conventional treatment for ADD and related syndromes involves taking a medicine called Ritalin, which is a central nervous system stimulant, essentially a form of speed, like Dexedrine, dextroamphetamine, or amphetamines. Over the last few decades, these kinds of drugs have been used to treat a variety of ailments. In the 1950s, Benzedrine inhalers were widely used to treat stuffy noses, which yield to this type of medicine just as they do to cocaine; that is, until a rebound effect causes nasal congestion, which is then relieved by another snort. Speed was also combined with aspirin and other painkillers to make effective remedies for menstrual cramps. Weight loss pills were based on amphetamines, like dexedrine. Many of us remember how effective these medications were, not only for losing weight but for staying up all night before an exam or for sharpening our wits for similar purposes. All these drugs became a significant problem for addiction-prone people in the 1950s and 1960s.

Ritalin is simply a variation on the molecule used in these drugs. Since 1990 there has been a 700 percent increase in the amount of Ritalin produced in the United States; nearly all of this increase can be ascribed to prescriptions for ADD.[3] Based on current trends, a conservative estimate is that 8 million American children will be taking Ritalin in the year 2000.[4]

I have no problem acknowledging that an occasional child—rare in my experience—responds to no other treatment and reacts so dramatically to modest doses of stimulants that it completely transforms his or her learning experience, making it a reasonable bargain. What does disturb me is that many doctors *routinely* prescribe this medication without investigating other possible causes for the child's behavior.

If the prescription of stimulant medications to large numbers of children is careless at best and knowing abuse at worst, what do I see as the solution to the problem? Let's consider an elegantly simple dietary intervention that brings about improvement in a significant percentage of the children I see. I'm not claiming that providing a high protein breakfast is the single remedy for attention deficit disorder or any other ailments. It is, however, a better way to begin to approach the problem and is part of my simple strategy to determine if a child is getting everything he should get and avoiding everything that may be disturbing him.

Children, just like adults, need to reinforce strong circadian rhythms. The shift from a conventional diet to one that emphasizes protein in the daytime and carbohydrates in the evening will accomplish this most effectively. The rules for the timing of protein and carbohydrate are simple, but the underlying chemistry is complicated. Of primary importance are the need to avoid morning carbohydrates because morning chemistry cannot handle them and the need to provide raw materials for the chemistry of consciousness, based as it is on a supply of amino acids from which we form the neurotransmitters needed for daytime vitality and alertness.

The Circadian Diet works for children with many different problems. I'm emphasizing attention deficit disorder and hyperactivity because they are so widespread. If your child has attention problems, the more closely he or she matches the following profile, the more likely he or she is to benefit from the diet.

- He or she doesn't eat breakfast.

- He or she eats sweetened cereal, fruit juices, jams and jellies, soda, sweet rolls, bagels, or white bread for breakfast.

- He or she craves carbohydrates at other meals and between meals.

- He or she sometimes or often appears drunk—sad, happy, silly, mean, or spacey drunk.

TRYING THE DIET WITH YOUR CHILD

If your child enjoys eating eggs and bacon or sausage, but you're worried about cholesterol and saturated fat, I suggest that you put aside your fears and allow him or her to load up on these foods at breakfast for a three-week period. The idea is to be practical and not fight over food if your child already likes such high protein and high fat foods. Once you have proven the point that a high protein breakfast of this kind improves your child's mood and performance, then you can consider alternatives that are lower in saturated fat for the long haul. At the same time, incorporate more protein into lunch and cut back on carbohydrates, saving them for the evening meal.

If eggs and bacon don't suit your child's tastes, then try the shake for breakfast. You can lace it with a sufficient amount of carbohydrate—strawberries, bananas, blueberries, or flavored yogurt—to make it palatable, if not downright tasty; the key is getting a strong morning dose of protein.

Some children refuse the shake. If that happens, you can experiment with shake popsicles. These were developed by Pamela Lamson, the mother of one of my patients. Her son Joey was a seriously autistic child. When I first saw him, he was in a total fog, living only on carbohydrates. He refused all protein, except for some milk, and was eating only frozen French fries, crackers, bread, pasta, and fruit. It was very difficult to get

Joey off the carbohydrates; he refused high protein foods and hated the shakes.

Joey's father David described the results produced by the shake popsicles like this: "Within three days of starting the shake popsicles Joey showed improvement in speech and eye contact, and he was much calmer. The proof in the pudding was that when Pamela took him off the popsicles (he had become constipated) he went hyper in two days. Within twelve hours of starting the popsicles again, Joey calmed down and returned to a much calmer and more focused state." A combination of the Circadian Diet and antifungal medicine for a yeast problem has changed Joey from someone lost in the deep chaos of autism to a sweet, verbal boy who is nearly on target developmentally.

SHAKE POPSICLES
(makes twelve small popsicles)

1 box or bag of frozen strawberries, thawed, or 2 pints of fresh strawberries

4 tablespoons soy protein powder

1 tablespoon flaxseed powder

2-4 tablespoons plain yogurt

⅔ cup water

1 box of strawberry-banana Jell-O gelatin

1. Pour thawed strawberries in the blender and add the protein powder, flaxseed powder, and yogurt. Boil the water and whisk in the Jell-O; add to mixture in the blender and blend well. If your child hates creamy textures and prefers an icier popsicle, omit the Jell-O and water.

2. Pour into popsicle molds. Freeze for several hours until firm. To unmold, hold popsicle under running hot water.

Even if your child rejects the shake at first, it is sufficiently edible to be the subject of negotiations and bribery long enough for both of you to see the benefits. I have a healthy respect for children's capacity to understand what a deal is, so I suggest that you explain it like this, with appropriate changes of wording if your child has a different problem, such as sleep disturbances, moodiness, or irritability: "Mickey, your teachers have noticed that you have a hard time paying attention, especially when you're bored. We know you're a smart kid, but you're going to find that if you can't pay attention to certain subjects, you're going to have trouble getting them under your belt. We think it may help to eat plenty of protein in the morning. If you like eggs, milk, beans, cheese, fish, or meat, you can have them for breakfast. Otherwise, we're going to make you a special milkshake. It doesn't taste bad, especially when it's mixed with strawberries, bananas, or other fruits you like. And if this helps you do better at school I think you'll agree it's a good deal."

Try the Circadian Diet with your child for three weeks. If it works beautifully and your child responds, that is all that's required. You can feel comfortable sticking with this diet indefinitely as a safe and sound approach to eating. If the diet makes a definite difference, but there's still room for improvement, or even if your child doesn't respond at all, you can take heart from the notion that what you're doing is healthy for him and that it's reasonable to continue the diet as part of good general nutrition.

TREAT THE CHILD, NOT JUST THE DISEASE

In medical school, I learned that there were distinct diseases that attacked people and that every illness had its own remedy. But my experience as a physician has led me to conclude that the same underlying conditions bring out different symptoms in different people. Whether your child fits easily into a diagnostic slot is not the issue; your focus should be treating your child, not the "disease."

When you work with children who have chronic illnesses, you soon understand that certain underlying issues come up repeatedly and that immune and biochemical imbalances head up the list. If you attend to these problems, you can get lots of children out of trouble with their health and behavior because the same solutions often work for children with different labels. Children with recurring ear infections, those who are frequently stuffy, wheezy, and sneezy, those who are constipated or have diarrhea, those who have irritated skin or an irritating personality and get under your skin, as well as those with attention problems and hyperactivity, may all benefit.

If your child hasn't responded sufficiently to the Circadian Diet, I suggest that you do some dietary detective work with your child in the hope of discovering whether some sort of imbalance or sensitivity is causing the problem. Every child is a unique individual, but this strategy may help any child overcome immune and biochemical imbalances that can be expressed in a dazzling variety of symptoms.

From my experiences with thousands of children, I've developed the following list of avenues to explore. The discovery and treatment of these conditions frequently leads to success. You may need the help of a cooperative physician in certain cases.

- Sensitivities to foods and substances in foods, such as additives and salicylates, has been a controversial issue for years. Even if the odds are only one in ten that your child has a problem caused or aggravated by sensitivities, it's worth checking out. A growing number of health professionals now agree that a diet that eliminates common allergenic foods and additives, such as sugars, dyes, milk, chocolate, potatoes, soy, pork, peanuts, tomatoes, apples, grapes, wheat, eggs, yeast, corn, and citrus may be extremely beneficial. The reliability of allergy testing varies considerably. I recommend a blood test for hidden delayed food allergies available from Immuno Laboratories. (Further information about the test is available at my Web site or from Immuno Laboratories in Fort Lauderdale, Florida, 1-800-231-9197.)

- Yeast problems, or the overgrowth of intestinal fungi as the result of taking antibiotics, aggravated by a high carbohydrate diet, can cause a wide variety of symptoms. (See chapter 8 for more information.)

- Magnesium deficiency or special needs for magnesium, especially in children with attention problems, hyperactivity, and tics—twitches of the face, neck, shoulders, eyes, or other body parts—is another common problem. I have seen numerous children in whom a diagnosis of Tourette's syndrome (a serious neurologic disorder in which tics are a feature) was mentioned by a consulting doctor on the basis of such twitches and tics. A simple magnesium supplement, such as 1 to 2 teaspoons per day of 18 percent magnesium solution from Cardiovascular Research, a supplement supplier, is often all that is needed to bring such symptoms under control.

- Problems with fatty acids, for the most part deficiencies of omega-3 oils, may affect anything from skin, hair, and nails to the functioning of the central nervous system. (For more information, see chapter 8.)

- Deficiencies of or special needs for calcium, zinc, B vitamins, and, for carbohydrate cravers, chromium can cause problems in body chemistry that result in different symptoms in different children. These children may respond to relatively large doses of vitamins and to normal doses of minerals. By itself, this particular approach to children's attention problems is not the most likely to give results in most children and should not take precedence over cleaning up a child's diet by providing fresh, varied, unrefined, additive-free food.

Although beyond the scope of this book, there is a longer list of factors, any one of which may be a bull's eye for your child. It includes everything from carbon monoxide poisoning to mold allergy to pinworms. For more information, see *The Hyperactivity Hoax,* by Dr. Sydney Walker.[5]

SOME CONSIDERATIONS FOR BABIES

Infants are born with their mothers' circadian rhythms, but the environment into which they are born puts them at high risk for losing this rhythm. Unlike that of grownups, babies' exposure to timegivers such as light, food, and social stimulation tends to favor disorganization. Babies are (and expect to be) fed frequently and tended to at all hours of the day and night, often with exposure to nighttime artificial light as part of the bargain.

It's crucial, then, to help them establish and maintain their own day and night cycle. Apart from eating, sleeping is a baby's main activity. Naturally, you want your baby to sleep at night and be awake as much as possible during the day. You can encourage this by appropriately timing exposure to stimulation and, most of all, to light. The trick to helping babies who are having trouble sleeping at night is to make sure that they have plenty of exposure to sunlight during the day and to darkness at night. Putting on a light in a baby's room in the middle of the night, even for a minute, can have a serious impact on her cyclic chemistry and deny her a chance to establish a solid day and night pattern.

After light, the most important factor in helping a baby establish circadian rhythm is entertainment. If your baby wakes at night needing to be fed or just wanting a little reassurance, I suggest that you do this with as little fuss as possible. Babies whose parents establish a firm pattern of having them sleep in a darkened room with minimal stimulation will learn that night is the time for sleep.

Most parents, however, experience a fundamental anxiety that translates into: "If I leave my baby alone in this room, he's going to die." Babies, perceptive creatures that they are, pick up on this and figure, "If she leaves me alone in this room, I'm going to die." As a parent, your main job is to help your child become a self-confident grownup; even babies must learn success and failure as well as develop a good sense of timing. So the message as you leave your baby's room should be: "Okay, Susie, I've swaddled you, I've nursed you, I've changed you, I've reassured you, and I know you're not sick because you just ate well. So now I'm going to put you down. I'm sure you'll be all right." The result may be a few minutes of screaming while the baby endures the panic of abandonment, but when she successfully overcomes that feeling, she will have achieved the ability to soothe herself and fall asleep. In a baby's world, conquering the perils of sleep is a major developmental victory, as well as an early contribution to the development of strong circadian rhythm. But here's a warning. After the age of two months, every month that you delay this confrontation will result in an extra hour of crying when you finally get around to it, and the battle may last for several days.

Although the timing of protein and carbohydrates is not relevant for babies, I would like to touch on one aspect of the Circadian Diet that does pertain to them—soy. I have been touting soy as an ideal food and a source of healthy protein and phytonutrients. You might then expect me to be strongly in favor of soy formula as a substitute for human, cow, or goat milk.

But I have my doubts about soy formula. Food contains information. No food contains as much information as milk. Human milk contains human information; cow's milk contains cow information; goat's milk contains goat information; and so on. There is no food that contains better information for babies than breast milk. Occasionally mother's milk carries citrus, yeast, or other allergens from the mother's diet that can disturb a baby. Except for this qualification, I strongly believe that mothers' milk is the best thing.

When formula feeding is a necessity rather than a preference and your baby can't tolerate cow's milk, soy formula becomes an option. In view of the potential of soy to modulate human hormone chemistry, might a soy-based formula have a downside? This issue has been studied with no clear resolution. According to a paper by Dr. Kenneth Setchell, a leading soy researcher, infants consuming soy-based formulas have an intake of hormonally active substances, when adjusted for body weight, of as much as ten times that of adults consuming soy foods.[6] And infants fed soy formula have been shown to have isoflavone plasma concentrations up to twenty thousand times higher than the hormone (estradiol) levels normally found in early life.[7] Even though the isoflavones are not really estrogens, such high concentrations certainly have the potential to produce unwanted effects. (Some scientists have expressed serious concern that hormones given to cattle that end up in our food supply and plasticizers that mimic estrogens provide developing children, as well as adults, with an overload of estrogen that increases cancer risk and results in developmental changes such as premature breast development in girls.) It remains possible that low, modest, or even high levels of soy intake may turn out to have long-term benefits for babies. But I remain wary, especially for babies who are consuming inappropriately large amounts of bottle feedings (more than 24 ounces per day).

Since intolerance to cow's milk is widespread, what can you choose, besides soy formula, if you cannot breastfeed your baby? There is no inexpensive answer, but I would recommend goat's milk, now readily available at health food stores. It's best if you can get certified fresh goat's milk. Be sure to provide a supplement of 50 micrograms of folic acid, in which goat's milk is curiously deficient. Your pediatrician can also recommend nonmilk, nonsoy formulas that are, unfortunately, rather costly. If you are currently feeding your baby soy formula, substitute goat's milk for half the feedings and keep the total amount of bottle fed formula and milk per day below 24 ounces. After nine months of age, begin to introduce solid foods, allowing them to make up an ever-increasing part of your baby's diet. And don't consider juice as a substitute; it's straight carbohydrates and could push your child into insulin resistance at an early age.

Americans carry a legacy that teaches a certain indifference to the connection between the quality of a child's diet and the child's ultimate health in adulthood. But beginning in infancy, a child's diet does have an impact on his health. You have control over what your infant eats. But as they get older, children can and do exercise a legitimate control over whether they will eat something. And your reluctance to change your child's diet may be multiplied when compounded by all the issues of nurture and rewards that embrace what families do with food. If I suggest that your child drink a protein shake with flaxseed powder in the morning, you may become entangled in a web of factors, including grandpa's need to slip him candy, grandma's worries that children can't grow without milk, and your child's objection that he can detect the intolerable texture of a few grains of flaxseed powder in a fifty-five-gallon drum of beverage.

Information is the best answer to the problem. (And bribery can be a big help.) You can propose a dietary change for your child as a brief experiment after which there will be some reward. One hopes that part of the reward will be the kinds of changes that Billy Malone experienced, clinching his commitment to the Circadian Diet.

On my taxi ride to be a guest on a talk show, my driver offered me this quote from an unknown source: "Love of country is the memory of the food we enjoyed as children." I'd add: Love of children can have no better expression than giving them happy memories associated with healthy food.

23:00
24:00
25:00
01:00
02:00
03:00
04:00
05:00
06:00
07:00
08:00
09:00
10:00
11:00
12:00
13:00
14:00
15:00
16:00
17:00
18:00
19:00
20:00
21:00
22:00
23:00
24:00
25:00
01:00

14

Men

My brother Dave wintered at McMurdo Sound in the Antarctic in 1955 as part of the Navy's Operation Deep Freeze. His was one of the first groups of human beings ever to deliberately spend the long, dark winter in Antarctica, where the sun sinks below the horizon in the fall and doesn't return until spring. The flip side of this period of prolonged night occurs during the summer, when the sun doesn't set.

Adding to the extraordinary circumstances of this expedition was the Navy's watch schedule, which consisted of four-hour shifts that rotated throughout a twenty-four-hour period, so that men might be up for duty at any time of day or night.

In the summer the men had to cope with constant daylight, so they were missing the normal cues to go to bed. "When it's daylight, even though it's midnight or one o'clock in the morning, you don't think of it as being the time to go to sleep," says Dave. "Your mind just says, hey, there's work to be done. I may be tired but I'm not recognizing the need for sleep because it's daylight."

Already lacking the strong time-giving effects of light, the men could not set their body clocks by what they were eating, either. "We had four meals a day. Two of them occurred at noon and midnight, the other two at six in the morning and six in the evening," continues Dave. "One of the difficulties in telling what time it was was that the 6:00 a.m. and 6:00 p.m. meals were powdered scrambled eggs, and the other two meals were stew. So if you woke up at six o'clock and went into the galley for a meal and you had powdered scrambled eggs, you didn't know whether you were having breakfast or dinner."

Despite losing the signals that are normally provided by the cycle of light and dark, the timing of activity, intake of food, reasonable work shifts, or even simple obedience to the clock, most of the men managed to get through without becoming acutely sick or injured. But some of them developed a condition they called Big Eye, in which they became stuck in a sleepless state. Almost everyone had duties that required exhausting physical labor, but even so, the men with Big Eye failed to sleep for days.

The men with Big Eye demonstrated that the body's flexibility is a double-edged sword. The loss of essential timegivers easily disrupted their circadian rhythms, probably setting them up for health problems if they continued down that path. On the other hand, proper application of some fairly simple rules for circadian health could have rescued them. And the same rules can rescue you from a potentially perilous state of disorganization.

The Circadian Prescription reinforces strong circadian rhythms; produces better sleep, enhanced moods, alertness, and energy; and reduces the risk for reproductive cancers for everyone. In addition to these overall improvements in health and well-being, there are specific aspects of the diet that have a favorable impact on prostate health, a subject that provokes anxiety for many men.

PROSTATE AILMENTS: THE "MALE PROBLEM"

There is certainly cause for concern. Prostate ailments are an almost universal threat to men in Europe and North America. Among men in the United States, prostate cancer is the most common cancer; it is also the second leading cause of cancer death.[1] In addition, countless men suffer from other prostate problems. This phenomenon represents a kind of "male problem" corresponding roughly to what used to be called "female problems," a much less specific collection of gynecological woes that were lumped under this heading in the mid-1900s. The notion of female problems embraced excessive menstruation, infertility, irregular periods, cramps, vaginal discharge, and other kinds of medical mischief that women endure.

The male problem is more localized in the prostate gland, the part of the male reproductive system that secretes fluids that help transport sperm. Nevertheless, it is a fairly complicated picture, which includes inflammations of the prostate, a common condition known as benign prostatic hypertrophy (BPH), and prostate cancer.

What's more, prostate problems may lead you to needing a cystoscopy, where a narrow flashlight is inserted into the hole from which you pee until it arrives in your bladder. On the way, it passes through your prostate gland. Cystoscopy is a procedure that causes "big eyes" in the bravest of men.

Besides cystoscopy, the other method often used to examine men with prostate complaints is digital rectal examination, in which the examiner can feel the profile of your prostate gland. (Digital refers to the doctor's finger, not his computer.) Both give much less information than you would expect to get from such relatively invasive procedures. Opening your mouth and saying "ah" discloses much more about your teeth, gums, tongue and throat than any rectal exam reveals about your prostate, unless you have a huge lump. Ultrasound, magnetic resonance imaging (MRIs), and computerized axial tomography (CAT) scans are necessary to get a good picture of what's happening to this gland, whose actual location on the floor of your pelvis seems mysterious to anyone who has not studied anatomy.

DIET AND PROSTATE HEALTH

If you look around you, especially as you get older and start hearing stories from men who have prostate trouble, you may wonder if there's something simple you can do to avoid it. I'm not talking about early detection, which is mentioned frequently these days. (Of course, most men's idea of early detection is that early next year or the year after would be just fine.) Nor am I saying that a good history, physical exam, measurements of prostate-specific antigen (PSA), a common blood test used to screen for prostate cancer, and other indicators of your underlying health, prostate or otherwise, are not a good idea.

But you're misplacing your priorities if you go through those procedures without making some modest changes in your diet now to prevent troubles in the future. Most men who have a reasonably healthy personal and family medical history and who don't abuse themselves with excesses of drugs, tobacco, and alcohol, other risky activities, or excessive inactivity can probably remain free of obvious symptoms even if they don't implement all the points of the Circadian Prescription. Some of these points are aimed at people who are trying to get out of serious medical trouble or who have risk factors that call on them to follow the diet very strictly.

Naturally, the more closely you follow the Circadian Prescription the better, but if you do nothing else, I urge you to consume soy protein and flaxseed powder daily to prevent prostate problems. By making these simple dietary changes and keeping your mind open to the possibility that fungal infection, intestinal overgrowth, or allergy might have a hand in any prostate inflammation that is not otherwise easily diagnosed by a physician, you can go a long way toward avoiding the possibility of getting prostate cancer, as well as the other problems that frequently lead men to undergo cystoscopy.

What I'm giving you here is a chance to climb the ship's mast with me so that from its top we can see far over the horizon of medicine. The view from the masthead is based not so much on my daily activities as a practicing physician but on my mission to search the seascape of scientific research for courses that can help prevent my patients from developing prostate trouble. What I see from the top of the mast is a body of evidence that is solid enough to support these simple changes in behavior, especially considering that there's zero risk in consuming flaxseed and soy protein.

The best evidence is based on studies done in a couple of places in the world where prostate troubles are rare. This work has been done by a number of people, including Dr. Herman Adlercreutz. A professor and multitalented researcher in Finland, Dr. Adlercreutz has conducted solid epidemiological studies that show a lower incidence of prostate cancer in men consuming foods popular among Finns and Chinese—rye bread for Finns and soy for Chinese.[2] And he has carried out elaborate chemical analyses and experiments to show which substances in these foods provide the protection.

For years before his research was done, it was assumed that the Finns' genetic history accounted for their lower incidence of prostate cancer. Most modern Finns come from a small number of people who migrated to that part of the world many years ago, so they are a rather distinct linguistic, racial, and genetic group. It turns out, however, that it's not their genes but their diet that protects them against certain cancers. And the dietary factor that is most significant is a sourdough rye bread that is eaten by people consuming a traditional Finnish diet. This whole-grain, heavy-duty bread is made out of ground whole rye seeds without anything removed. The leavening is provided by lactobacillus (acidophilus) instead of yeast, which is used to leaven almost all bread consumed in other parts of the world. What's key is that the rye fiber contains lignans that modulate hormone chemistry and reduce the risk of reproductive cancers.

RYE BREAD: THE FINNISH SOLUTION

You don't have to live in Finland to try this bread. You can order it from a bakery in Canada which ships it UPS. (Dimpflmeier Bakery, 1-800-724-6636.) I keep it in my freezer until I'm ready to eat it. Consuming two slices of this bread daily is another way you can fight prostate problems. But it is relatively high in carbohydrate content, so you should consume it in the evening.

23:00
24:00
25:00
01:00
02:00
03:00
04:00
05:00
06:00
07:00
08:00
09:00

Dr. Adlercreutz and others have also done experiments to show that flaxseed contains more lignans than rye fiber; in fact, there's no other food that even approaches flaxseed when it comes to lignan content.

Flax is described in detail in chapter 3. Eastern Europeans have traditionally used flaxseeds as a source of food and medicine. Flaxseed oil, which makes up about one-third of the weight of the seeds, has extremely healthy properties that also provide particular benefits for the prostate gland. But here we're talking about the *fiber* in the flaxseed. The best way to use the seeds is to grind them in a coffee mill. You can then consume the fine, fluffy powder as part of a shake or add it to a variety of other foods. Your aim is to eat a heaping tablespoon per day.

Besides rye and flaxseed, there are other foods that contain lignans. Some of the best sources include legumes (especially lentils, kidney, fava, and navy beans), seeds (like sunflower seeds), seaweed, cereal brans, and whole grains.

There is also a solid body of evidence supporting the role of soy protein in reducing the risk of prostate cancer. For example, research has shown that isoflavones, substances contained in soybeans, modify testosterone metabolism, decreasing the risk for both benign prostatic hypertrophy and prostate cancer.[3] Incorporating soy protein in your diet doesn't require you to change what you eat, although it's fine to eat more tofu, miso, and other soy products if you enjoy them. The simplest, quickest way to consume soy protein is by stirring soy protein isolate, a relatively tasteless substance, into some of the food you are already eating.

Foods like soybeans, flaxseed, and rye contain information derived from phytonutrients, which keep animals in synchrony with the rhythm of the seasons and which have profound effects on our own reproductive systems (see chapter 3).

Prostate Inflammation, or Nonspecific Prostatitis

Your prostate gland usually doesn't speak to you until it's in some advanced state of trouble. When it does, it has only two voices. One is expressed through pain or difficulty with urination, and the other is just plain pain, which is almost invariably felt in the midline of your body. The spectrum of difficulties includes inflammation, enlargement, and cancer. While there are more or less pure representations of each one, the lines between them are often blurred. All three, but particularly enlargement and cancer, are addressed by the preventive measures included in the Circadian Diet.

Let's start with inflammation, which is the medical term for some combination of redness, pain, swelling, and heat that almost always accompanies infection but may also represent your body's reaction to noninfectious irritants or allergens. The flame of prostate inflammation is experienced as burning with urination. This is as much a result of inflammation of the tube through which the urine passes out of the penis (the urethra) as it is due to inflammation of the prostate, per se, which lies astride this tube, just beneath the bladder. Germs that infect the urethra, such as the gonorrhea germ, may ascend it and get into the prostate gland. There, the alkaline environment and blood supply, which are conducive to bacterial growth, make it much harder to treat the infection with antibiotics than, say, a sore throat, a boil, or an uncomplicated pneumonia. Because the germs that infect the prostate are difficult to extract from a patient for a culture it has become a common practice for doctors to treat symptoms of prostate inflammation with antibiotics without knowing what germ, if any, might be there.

The diagnosis in this situation is "nonspecific" prostatitis, which is a well-accepted medical term. But when you stop to think about it, it's peculiar. According to medical principles, when there is an infection, the perpetrator is almost always a particular germ. The prostate, like all internal tissues, is not likely to be infected by more than one germ at a time. The implication is that if there's an infection, it's quite specific. How then do we come up with the diagnosis "nonspecific" prostatitis? It's a result of several factors; efforts to recover a germ are to no avail, the prostate acts as if there's an inflammation—with swelling, pain, difficulty urinating, and sometimes cloudy or pussy urine—and antibiotics are at least temporarily soothing. But after antibiotic treatment, this problem recurs more often than other infections.

What happened with my patient Brooks shows how this scenario plays out. It also reveals why I think that such mysterious and sometimes chronic inflammations of the prostate are usually not infections but instead have a lot to do with factors that are also related to abnormal growth or cancers of the prostate.

Brooks is a fifty-year-old businessman whose previously dependable penis had become much less reliable with regard to its sexual responsibilities. At the same time he suffered from discomfort with urination, some hesitancy in starting his urinary stream, and the need to get up at night to urinate more than once, which had been his previous custom. He was alarmed that whatever was going on represented some sort of permanent equipment failure. Told at first by both a general practitioner and a urologist that his prostate was "pretty normal" and later that it was a "little enlarged," he had undergone two courses of antibiotic treatment for nonspecific prostatitis. His symptoms improved while he was on the antibiotics but returned when he finished the medication.

I had a telephone consultation with him, and after hearing him out and considering various possibilities, I suggested to him that he had "some kind of mischief" with his prostate. This was a much softer diagnosis than that of nonspecific prostatitis. But it suggested a treatment that was aimed more at making his prostate happy than at trying to kill some unseen, unidentified, and perhaps nonexistent germs.

The concept of trying to make some organ in your body happy seems alien to a regular guy like Brooks. He shares with most people the medical notion that there is a specific treatment for every condition and that this treatment is not a strategy to make some part of your body happy. It did, however, make Brooks happy when I suggested that part of his therapy was at least daily efforts to encourage the emptying of his prostate and its tubing by provoking an ejaculation. This was contrary to the no-sex advice he had been given earlier, which seemed to me like the equivalent of telling someone with a bad cold not to blow his nose.

I offered Brooks a package of additional measures to make his prostate happy. These included daily doses of soy protein, flaxseed powder, flaxseed oil, zinc, and an antifungal medicine. If you understand why I loaded my shotgun with such a diversity of remedies and how they all fit together, you will also see how I perceive that the whole range of prostate mischief from inflammation to cancer fits together.

I've already explained the soy protein and flaxseed powder. I also recommended an additional supplement of flaxseed oil. The prostate gland is one of the richest sources of the hormonelike substances that are made from omega-3 fatty acids, with which flaxseed oil is loaded. They are called prostaglandins, named for the very organ under discussion, because they were first isolated from fluids found in the prostate. (Soon after their discovery in prostatic fluids, they were found to be present in a wide variety of animal tissues of all kinds and not at all exclusive to the prostate, but the name stuck.) The use of fatty acids in flaxseed oil helps the prostate make prostaglandins. But the more important motive for a prescription of flaxseed oil was the strong likelihood that Brooks, like most people, was deficient in omega-3 oils. The flaxseed oil, then, was generally beneficial rather than a treatment aimed specifically at the prostate.

I recommended that Brooks take zinc because it helps the immune system fight off infections and control the body's inflammatory response to infection. Finally, I prescribed the antifungal medicine because of my consistent experience with other patients where I'd seen that an overgrowth of fungus germs, particularly yeasts, has a proclivity to bother people's reproductive systems. I have often found stubborn cases of prostate problems in men to be responsive to antifungal drugs.

But there's another, more important angle to the antifungal treatment I gave Brooks and the many other men I've treated in a similar way. In order for the isoflavones and lignans in soy protein and flaxseed powder to be transformed into the substances that beneficially modulate hormone chemistry, they must pass through the digestive tract, where they are changed by certain germs that live there. If the normal distribution of healthy flora has been disturbed so that there are too many bad germs and not enough good germs, the capacity of the intestinal flora to help hormone chemistry will be seriously impaired. Antibiotics are by far the most significant disrupter of intestinal germ populations. A single course of an antibiotic prescription can affect this balance for months or longer. (See chapter 8 for more information.) My prescription of an antifungal medicine for Brooks was aimed at two overlapping targets. One was the possibility that a fungal infection was directly related to the prostate inflammation; the other was that his two courses of antibiotics had made him worse by causing a disturbance in his bowel germ population that would correct itself once the number of yeast germs living there was reduced.

Within ten days Brooks and his prostate were both happy. His equipment returned to reliable functioning, and he has remained well since. He is as pleased as he is surprised. This is true for many men whose similar responses to simple changes in diet don't jibe with their expectation that I would have to treat them by calling out the big guns rather than coaxing their bodies back into balance. I'm confident that the remedies I suggested for Brooks worked because they were specifically connected to achieving a hormonal balance governed by a combination of factors related to his digestive flora and an intake of substances that made his prostate happy.

It's not a big step from consideration of acute problems, such as what Brooks had, to the more chronic problems of prostate enlargement and prostate cancer.

BENIGN PROSTATIC HYPERTROPHY AND PROSTATE CANCER

Benign prostatic hypertrophy is an enlargement of the prostate that's called benign because it is not due to cancer cells. Still, the enlargement can be far from benign if it results in a lack of control over functions that we all take for granted, including urinating when you want to urinate and only then. A single urinary accident in front of your classmates in the first grade can constitute a major, unforgettable scar in one's childhood; a repeat performance, like that of my sixty-year-old patient while standing in line at the check-in counter at O'Hare Airport, is no joke either. Nor is "benign" the right word to describe the condition that underlies such loss of control. BPH may also involve getting up frequently at night to urinate, with the intense urgency to do so unfortunately combined with a disconcerting hesitancy of performance and a lack of reward in the volume of urine produced.

Although the symptoms of BPH can be severe, it is ironic that men with prostate cancer often have no symptoms. As they age, most men, on biopsy, show signs of prostate cancer. In fact, by the time they are in their eighties, nearly all men have prostate cancer, as defined by the typical cancerous appearance of cells under the microscope. Yet, because this particular cancer grows slowly and spreads infrequently, only a small percentage of men actually become sick or die from the disease. (A man's lifetime risk of dying from prostate cancer is a little less than 3 percent.)[4]

Given the low odds of illness or death from prostate cancer, it's confusing from a medical standpoint when a sixty-, seventy- or eighty-year-old man has a prostate biopsy and is found to have cancer cells. Because the question of the actual malignancy of the condition—how likely it is that the cancer will grow quickly enough to cause problems—is difficult to resolve, it encourages a more aggressive approach to therapy than might otherwise be warranted. Since aggressive therapy frequently involves either removing testicles or taking female hormones, which can produce dramatic changes in a man's body, this is not a trivial question.

Natural therapies for treating or, more important in the context of this chapter, preventing illness are not usually studied in the same way as pharmaceuticals, because no one can patent a naturally occurring substance like flaxseed powder and make enough money to justify the enormous expense of carefully conducted, controlled, and double-blinded studies. Still, the studies by Dr. Adlercreutz mentioned earlier clearly show that consuming soy protein and other isoflavone and lignan-containing foods reduces the risk of prostate cancer. And the cancer data suggest strongly—and there is abundant anecdotal evidence to support it—that the same hormonal environment that leads to the high incidence of cancer in older men in our culture, but not in Chinese and Finnish men, is also associated with the risk for prostatic enlargement.[5]

The simple strategy for preventing the range and frequency of prostate problems is to consume more soy protein, flaxseed powder, and rye fiber. If you happen to be a regular bacon, ham, or sausage and eggs kind of guy, I urge you to substitute the shake, with its soy protein and flaxseed powder, at least four days a week. It's good that you're eating protein at your morning meal and getting the lift you need at the beginning of the day, but what you're eating will not protect your health like soy protein and flaxseed. (If you don't have time for breakfast, see the section for travelers in the appendix, where you'll find a quick shortcut that will help you get your soy protein and flaxseed every day.)

THE CIRCADIAN DIET AND HEART DISEASE: IT'S NOT JUST THE CHOLESTEROL

Coronary heart disease (CHD) is the number one killer of both men and women in the United States. Each year, more than five hundred thousand Americans die of heart attacks caused by CHD. Soy intake has been shown to lower cholesterol and decrease cardiovascular disease associated with high cholesterol. There is growing scientific evidence to support this; for example, one recent study showed that a diet high in soy protein reduced cholesterol by as much as 20 percent.[6] Other research has demonstrated that soy protein lowers triglycerides and reduces the oxidation of LDL, or "bad" cholesterol, which contributes to blood vessel problems linked to cardiovascular disease.[7] And flaxseed has also been shown to lower both total and LDL cholesterol.[8] The Circadian Diet, which includes daily intake of soy protein and flaxseed powder, ensures that you get this important protection.

But cholesterol is not the exclusive evil agent in heart disease. Some people, especially those with complicating conditions of diabetes, tobacco smoking, and a strong family history of heart disease and obesity, carry cholesterol-related risks. But most people who have heart attacks and other complications of "hardening of the arteries" have fairly normal cholesterol levels.

The tide of medical thinking is changing when it comes to heart disease. It looks as if issues related to carbohydrate excess, insulin resistance, and homocysteine and its control by folic acid will take center stage away from cholesterol.[9] The benefits of substances like flaxseed and soy are not due solely to lowering cholesterol. Soy and flaxseed do indeed lower serum cholesterol, but they also modify carbohydrate and fat metabolism, further decreasing your cardiovascular risk. You don't have to be taking aim at your cholesterol to get benefits from soy, flaxseed, and the Circadian Diet.

Like many men, you may have a tendency not to think about your health, shrugging off warnings from your mother, spouse, doctor, and children as well as newspapers and television programs that try to scare or educate you about activities that are dangerous to your well-being. Nor do you want to listen to me when I say that failure to adhere to basic circadian principles may eventually show up as something noticeably wrong with your health. But my advice in this chapter is simple: there are some painless things you can do to reap what are potentially major rewards for your long-term health.

24:00
25:00
01:00
02:00
03:00
04:00
05:00
06:00
07:00
08:00
09:00
10:00
11:00
12:00
13:00
14:00
15:00
16:00
17:00
18:00
19:00
20:00
21:00
22:00
23:00
24:00
25:00
01:00

CHAPTER

15

Chronic Illness

When I explain the detective work I use to unravel my patient's problems, I sometimes enumerate the "Tacks Laws" to illustrate my point. Keep them in mind as you set about the task of treating your chronic illness. There are two:

- It takes a lot of aspirin to feel good when you are sitting on a tack.

    No matter what you use for relief—aspirin, massage, vitamins, or meditation—the best treatment for sitting on a tack is removing the tack. In other words, don't just cover up a symptom; instead, get at the root of a problem by discovering its cause.

- If you are sitting on two tacks, removing only one does not necessarily make you feel 50 percent better.

    Chronic illnesses are frequently the result of a web of interrelated factors. Your body may be reacting to a germ, an allergen, or a toxin or you may be deficient in a vital nutrient. And the whole situation may be complicated by insulin resistance. It's unrealistic to think that finding and treating just one piece of the puzzle will be sufficient to remedy the problem. Restoring balance is a more realistic approach.

BALANCE AND HEALTH

Balance is a key concept in most alternative medical approaches to health, such as traditional Chinese medicine, naturopathy, homeopathy, and Ayurveda. One of the problems that mainstream medicine has with these alternative medical systems is that the practitioners appear to offer the same remedy for all sorts of illnesses. This doesn't seem right to doctors trained to think that there are a certain number of discrete diseases that exist in nature. Physicians have also been taught that for each disease there is a *distinct* treatment. We know, for example, that if you have a strep throat or pneumonia a particular antibiotic is the right treatment, while another antibiotic is appropriate for your urinary tract infection because a different germ is involved. If you burn your finger or you break your arm, the treatment is again going to be designed for the specific problem that you have.

There is certainly some truth to the idea that specific illnesses or conditions need precise, individualized treatments. But there is another valid argument to be made as we move away from acute ailments to focus on the increasing prevalence of chronic illnesses. Sometimes the symptoms of a chronic illness can be suppressed with drugs, but since the cause of the disease is unknown, an individualized remedy to cure the person is out of the question. When an alternative medical practitioner recommends a generalized strategy that is not necessarily aimed at the distinct disease but is more directed at correcting imbalance, these approaches are designed to get to the underlying causes rather than the individual symptoms.

If you are in pain, it's hard to believe in a treatment unless it works right away. Dietary changes and other generalized strategies, like the Circadian Prescription, usually do not produce *instant* relief. These measures do sometimes take effect quickly, but it's frequently a slower process. I think you will be more motivated if you understand what lies behind much chronic illness.

RHYTHMIC DISTURBANCES MAY UNDERLIE
MANY CHRONIC ILLNESSES

As researchers continue to elucidate the mysteries of the scientific basis of disease, we realize more and more that similar fundamental mechanisms underlie much chronic illness. These include abnormalities of cell membranes and their capacity to send and receive messages, the backfiring of chemistry designed for cellular defense (autoimmunity and inflammation) and "sparks" from your own metabolic fire, environmental radiation, and chemical pollutants (oxidative damage). This is why a generalized strategy to treat chronic illness is beneficial.

To this list I would add dyschronism, or the failure to keep the various cadences of the body's biochemical activities in harmony. Disharmony is the direct cause of jet lag, symptoms related to shift work, and some sleep disturbances. But having your body in disharmony is also likely to bring out the worst in you more readily than if your body is well tuned. Poor tuning contributes indirectly to the expression of other illnesses, as indicated by the tendency for many ailments to have their own characteristic time peak of maximum intensity. There is evidence to support the idea that there is a rhythmic component in a number of diseases; among the most significant findings related to dyschronism are the following:[1]

- Seasonal affective disorder is a form of depression directly linked to the shorter daylight hours of winter.

- Sudden cardiac death and nonfatal heart attacks occur most frequently between 7:00 and 11:00 a.m.

- Strokes occur more frequently between 6:00 a.m. and noon.

- Asthma sufferers experience their worst symptoms in the early morning hours.

- The growth of breast cancer cells may be inhibited by melatonin. (When a 1995 study showed that Finnish flight attendants had an increased risk of breast cancer, the principal investigator hypothesized that frequently crossing time zones was part of the problem, since jet lag interferes with the normal production of melatonin. Although his theory has not yet been proven, other studies have shown that melatonin inhibits the growth of breast cancer cells.)

- Circadian rhythms have been substantiated in the symptoms of rheumatoid arthritis (least pain and stiffness around 5 p.m.) and allergic rhinitis (peak of worst symptoms between 5:00 and 7:00 a.m.).

CHRONIC INFLAMMATORY ILLNESS AND INSULIN RESISTANCE

Allowing for the fact that genetics affects an individual's susceptibility to disease, the roots of chronic illness often lie in deficiencies of various nutrients, other dietary issues, and hypersensitivity to foods and environmental factors, such as toxins. Whichever of these factors apply to you or your family, insulin resistance may be the easiest to recognize and correct. When you have this condition (if necessary, you can refer to the Insulin Resistance Checklist in chapter 4) high levels of insulin, created by frequent intake of carbohydrates, spill over into biochemical injury that makes whatever you have worse. This can include asthma, eczema, colitis, depression, headaches, psoriasis and much more.

What is common to all of these problems is inflammation. Whether you're looking under the microscope or studying its basic chemical reactions, inflammation is the same, wherever it's found. Chronic cough and mucus; sore, swollen, stiff joints; cramps and diarrhea; a chronically red, itchy rash; or periodontal disease—all are inflammation. Even cardiovascular disease, which used to be called hardening of the arteries and is now called atherosclerosis, is recognized as a fundamentally inflammatory process.

The first step in the biochemistry of inflammation is the release of informational substances from injured cells that attract the attention of healing mechanisms, the way a phone call to the automobile club brings you roadside assistance. The aid mobilized by these cellular calls for repair work is usually limited to the immediate task at hand; it's designed for mending a cut or recovering from a burn or fighting infection. But if the agent causing the inflammation persists or if something goes wrong with the signaling mechanisms involved in the call for help, the repair work and its accompanying signals (pain, swelling, redness, and heat) may become stuck, leaving you with a chronic inflammation. Chronic inflammatory diseases are often described by medical terms that end in "itis" and "osis."

Because the signaling mechanisms involved in chronic inflammation may be distorted by inappropriately high insulin levels in your body, this

CARBOHYDRATE CRAVING AND INSULIN RESISTANCE

After asking people about their eating habits for the last thirty years it's hard for me to say the word "carbohydrate" and not follow it with the word "craving." So what is it that gets you out of your chair at 9:00 p.m., after you've already eaten a good dinner, and compels you to the refrigerator or the cookie jar? And why do you choose to devour what you do?

Unlike other kinds of cravings—for salt or minerals, for example, which are right on target, urging you to eat exactly what your body needs—craving starchy and sugary foods is so off target that the target is you. What should be a self-protective instinct turns into self-destructive behavior. If you have a wicked carbohydrate craving, insulin resistance is likely to be a feature in the landscape of your health.

Rule number 1 when our ancestors hunted for food was: If it tastes sweet, it has sugar in it. Anything you find in nature that has a sweet taste is good to eat—that is, not poisonous—and contains sugars, which are a friendly source of carbohydrate. (There may be one tiny exception, which is the herb stevia; its apparent sweetness is not from sugar.)

Common sense, as well as experiments with babies, teaches us that the human yen for sweet-tasting substances is inborn to a certain extent. But craving is different from this basic mild preference for sweet-tasting substances. It goes way beyond an aptitude for selecting what is edible. Craving is a modification, even a perversion, of innate preferences.

The perversion goes like this (see chapter 4 for more detail). Given the equipment that you've inherited from your ancestors, you're inclined to increase your insulin levels when you eat carbohydrates. If you eat them frequently, your insulin levels become ratcheted up bit by bit until they get hung up on a relatively high level. When this occurs, the high levels of insulin quickly sweep sugar out of your bloodstream, signaling your brain that there is a sugar shortage.

What you feel is not hunger, which is what you feel after not eating for a long time. Carbohydrate craving is a sure sign that carbohydrates are exactly what you shouldn't eat if you want to stop the spiral of craving, insulin release, and more craving. On the other hand, you are supposed to eat carbohydrates for energy. The way out of this dilemma is to bring down your insulin levels by eating carbohydrates only in the evening.

is something over which you have control. Controlling insulin levels through appropriate dietary changes, including reducing carbohydrate consumption or shifting most consumption of carbohydrates to the later part of the day, will result in a positive effect on the biochemistry of inflammation. Although this dietary change is not directed at a specific disease, it should be part of any comprehensive treatment since it is aimed at easing the predictably disordered chemistry of anyone with a chronic inflammatory illness.

Medications that simply squelch the inflammation may not always be the best course of treatment. Granted, there are instances in which the cause is long gone but the body has gotten stuck in some kind of inappropriate reaction. In these cases, subduing the symptoms temporarily may work. But it's different when it comes to the daily, long-term application of steroid creams or the consumption of systemic steroids or anti-inflammatory drugs. These treatments have some fairly dreadful gastrointestinal side effects, including the tendency to create leaks in the intestinal walls that allow the entry of unwanted toxins, chemicals, and allergens into the bloodstream.

THE CIRCADIAN PRESCRIPTION FOR TREATING CHRONIC ILLNESS

Chronic illness makes you listen to your body. The message is not so precise that you know exactly what to change, unless of course it's something like chronic cough in a smoker. Most of the time, chronic pain or other signs of inflammation don't announce their cause. They demand that you do some detective work, presumably with the help of a professional who has good instincts and expertise at reading your body's communications by carefully listening to your story, interpreting laboratory tests, and then making educated efforts at trial and error.

Anyone with a chronic illness has to be especially aware of the second Tacks Law: if you are sitting on two tacks, removing only one does not necessarily make you feel 50 percent better. This means that insulin resistance is just one of many manageable factors that may also include improving other aspects of nutritional status and looking for the trigger, irritant, allergen, toxin, or germ to which your body may be responding.

Doing the detective work required to find underlying triggers of a chronic illness may take a long time; nor is it always successful. As a more generalized strategy, the ten steps of the Circadian Prescription (summa-

FOOD CRAVINGS AND ALLERGIES

Allergic craving is an important example of how mistaken is the myth that people, especially children, know what's good for them. "Is there any food that you crave or consume daily?" is an indispensable question in my patient interviews. The answer frequently leads to the discovery of a food allergy. Because it belies common sense, I often have to overcome my patient's protests by explaining that allergic individuals often control their symptoms by eating too much of the very food that troubles them. The immune system is so overwhelmed by the excess of whatever substance usually calls up the allergic reaction that the reaction itself is subdued. The phenomenon, called masking, gives the lie to the statement: "It couldn't be the orange juice, doc, because I drink it every day." Of course, that's precisely the point.

23:00
24:00
25:00
01:00
02:00
03:00
04:00
05:00
06:00
07:00
08:00
09:00
10:00
11:00
12:00
13:00
14:00
15:00
16:00
17:00
18:00
19:00

rized in the next chapter) will not only prevent or tame insulin resistance, a major contributor to chronic illness, but will reinforce healthy body rhythms and foster rhythmic integration. Remember that flexibility is your body's treasure; it enables you to be more like an orchestra, with its constant active effort to stay in tune and on beat, than a mechanical system. The same flexibility that allows you to fall victim to the negative effects of poorly timed eating, breathing, exercise, or exposure to light also permits you to use such influences for your benefit.

VISUALIZATION AND CHRONIC DISEASE

To the ten steps of the Circadian Prescription, I'd suggest adding visualization, another powerful tool for controlling chronic disease. Life consists of moving forward into images. You get to the dry cleaners to pick up your laundry by making a mental picture of the journey and moving forward into that picture. No picture, no laundry. With visualization, you are going to create an inner picture in order to realize your intention, not just in the outside world of the dry cleaner but in the inside world of your immune system.

The first step is to get the knack of meditation so that your mind and body are in a receptive posture for visualization (see chapter 10). Let's assume that you've learned to enter a meditative state; riding on the letter M, your mind can enter a new space within your consciousness. From here, you can take one step forward into your imagination and make a picture of what you want to accomplish in your body.

The effectiveness of this approach was initially proven in an experiment conducted with doctors suffering from terminal or advanced cancer. They were shown accurate images of their own cancer cells and of their immune system cells and were asked to create a realistic visualization of the immune system cells attacking the cancer cells. Most of the doctors successfully curbed their cancer—not to the extent of actually curing it, but in most cases there was measurable improvement. Since then, numerous experiments have shown that a less accurate image of the enemy is just as effective.[2]

About twenty years ago I used to meet one evening every month with a group of other doctors, including Dr. Bernie Siegel, one of the pioneers of visualization. Bernie shared fascinating examples of the kinds of imagery cancer patients chose to promote healing of their illnesses. It seemed important that the image be accurate in its intent; it was disconcerting when patients chose wimpy defensive images that were the imaginary equivalent of trying to beat their cancer with a wet noodle. People who chose aggressive images did better; lions, tigers, sharks, polar bears, and knights in shining armor do better work than a little girl gathering up cancer cells into snowballs and throwing them over the fence.

But what's a good image if you have chronic inflammatory disease? In this case, redness, heat, swelling, and pain afflict some part of your body as it reacts to an enemy that the doctor hasn't been able to discover or that has disappeared from the scene of the crime, leaving your immune system in a perpetual dither. You need a picture that is soothing but not self-defeating by way of quieting your immune reactions to the point of defenselessness. This is where a chemical or an abstract image may be more appropriate. By chemical image, I mean something along the lines of "Let's put out the fire." Remember that inflammation is an expression of your body's fire burning out of control. Whether it is in the skin, the digestive tract, the lungs, the heart, the nose, or the eyes or, for that matter, whether or not it is producing palpable heat, some kind of uncontrolled fire is at the bottom of a lot of chronic illness. Parkinson's disease, for example, has been characterized as a fire in the brain. And the oxidative damage in the chemistry of autistic children constitutes a kind of fiery injury to their RNA and DNA.

If you are going to employ visual imagery to quench the fire, then why not use pictures that are more effective than merely aiming a fire hose or throwing ice water at it? Instead, try mobilizing your body's powerful natural resources for quenching the inflammation, calling on your body's clouds to release rainwater on the brush fires of the prairie where the inflammation resides. This could be your intestine if you have colitis, your joints if you have arthritis, your skin if you have dermatitis, your lungs if you have bronchitis, and so on. You can even get technical and make your raindrops into vitamin C, vitamin E, beta-carotene, and other potent antioxidants. Communication between your meditating-visualizing brain and the resources of your body is more dynamic and more specific then you know.

When Bernie Siegel began talking about people's responsibility for their own health and healing in the face of serious illnesses such as cancer, people accused him of "blaming the victim" by placing an unreasonable burden of guilt on the sick person. But you can't really take control of your health without believing that your health is to some extent under your control. Even a person who has been a victim of some catastrophic accident must believe that he or she can exercise control over healing, to at least a small but critical degree, through the expression of intention in prayer or visualization or by the exercise of sheer willpower.

For people with chronic illness the lines of causation are more ambiguous than they are in an accident. However irrational it may be, all of us feel guilt for things that happen, like the ill-timed flareup of cold sores just before an important public appearance. Feeling guilty won't get you anywhere, but feeling responsible is the key to taking charge. If you feel like you're the passive victim of the event, you may miss a chance to engage your body's resources for healing. Only by feeling that you can take responsibility for your own health will you be able to make the changes that are necessary for regaining that health in the face of chronic illness.

24:00
25:00
01:00
02:00
03:00
04:00
05:00
06:00
07:00
08:00
09:00
10:00
11:00
12:00
13:00
14:00
15:00
16:00
17:00
18:00
19:00
20:00
21:00
22:00
23:00
24:00
25:00
01:00

Conclusion: The Ten Steps
of the Circadian Prescription

M ost of us are not as afraid of death as we are of dependency and a painful, expensive decline. Medical opinion on this subject has shifted away from the idea that aging and illness invariably go together, thanks partly to the work of Dr. James Fries. Some years ago, he began writing about the "rectangularization of the morbidity curve."[1] The idea is simple: to stay as healthy and fit as possible until we die rather than tumbling down a slippery slope of ill health beginning in our youth or middle age.

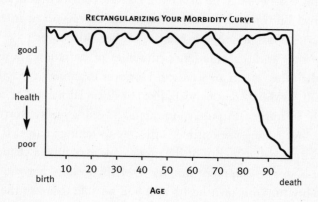

RECTANGULARIZING YOUR MORBIDITY CURVE

Along the bottom on the left side is your birth, and on the right is your death. At the top is good health, and at the bottom is illness. Rectangularizing your morbidity curve means staying at the top of the rectangle, where your health is good, from birth until death, rather than the lower, more painful diagonal road to the inevitable outcome that awaits us all.

His more recent publication provides good validation that his notion is not just an interesting idea.[2]

Dr. Fries's work has shown that people who take steps toward balance in their lives can age without illness to a much greater extent than was previously thought possible. Rhythms are not the focus of his work; however, I believe that rhythms—the natural rhythms of the earth, the circadian rhythms of your body, and the interconnectedness of your body's various rhythms, or rhythmic integration—are key to maintaining balance and robust health.

Throughout this book, I've explained how to reinforce healthy circadian rhythms and achieve rhythmic integration. The ten steps of the Circadian Prescription that follow don't take much time or many resources but they go a long way toward helping you stay healthy if you are well or feel better if you are ill.

1. Follow the Circadian Diet. Put protein in your morning meal, snacks, and lunch, either by drinking the Rhythmic Shake or by emphasizing high protein foods. Move most of your carbohydrates from breakfast, lunch, and morning snacks to the evening.

2. If you scored high on the insulin resistance test in chapter 4, adhere as rigorously as you can to the Circadian Diet. Because insulin resistance is at the root of so many conditions, you want to capitalize on your ability to bring down your serum insulin level. Eat the maximum tolerable amount of your protein during the day and save as many of your carbohydrates as possible for one meal in the evening. Craving carbohydrates is your enemy in this regard; you will probably need to make a gradual transition to the level of strictness that I'm recommending. That way, your insulin levels will come down step by step; they will not be screaming for carbohydrates while I'm screaming at you not to eat them.

3. Excess alcohol and caffeine interfere with circadian rhythm. The definition of excess depends on the person and on the time of day. In the early evening, the effects of alcohol are minimized by most people's capacity to easily metabolize 2 to 4 ounces of liquor over a two- to four-hour period. But efficient alcohol

metabolism declines dramatically after 10:00 p.m., making late night drinking particularly disruptive. Avoid caffeine except at around 4:00 p.m., the one time of day when its circadian effects are neutral.

4. Stay away from diet drinks because they send a false signal to your body. They promise the potential arrival of sugar and then, after engaging your body's mechanism for raising insulin, let you down when the sugar doesn't arrive.

5. Get plenty of full spectrum sunlight in your eyes and on some part of your skin every day. When you expose your eyes to sunlight—and I hope it's obvious that I don't mean staring at the sun—do it without wearing spectacles. These days spectacles of all kinds block both the healthy and the injurious types of ultraviolet rays. So get out in the sun, take off your glasses, and soak up a moderate amount of sunlight—at least one-half hour near dawn or dusk—every day. This does not require sunbathing, simply being out in the sun. If you live in a northern latitude where the winter days are short and there are lots of rainy, snowy, or cloudy days, then consider getting a light box like those prescribed for people with seasonal affective disorder. Expose yourself to the light box for at least a couple of hours every day.

6. Establish a regular time for going to bed at night and getting up in the morning and get sufficient sleep every night, preferably during the natural period of darkness between sundown and sunrise. While you're asleep, expose yourself to light as little as possible. If you wake up in the middle of the night to pee, don't turn on the light. Instead, use a dim flashlight or nightlight to light your way to the bathroom. Even a tiny amount of light at night will squash your melatonin peak. Remember that melatonin is an antioxidant and informational substance whose narrowly timed peak in the middle of the night, following a healthy exposure to light during the day, may be suppressed by ill-timed light. Failure to have a peak release of melatonin at night is like missing a bus that comes only once a day.

7. Encourage rhythmic harmony by learning to breathe with your diaphragm. When you relinquish control to your diaphragm, your breathing will take on the normal rhythm directed by the unconscious part of your brain rather than the potentially asynchronous rhythm generated by your chest muscles. This works especially well when you engage in stressful activities that make you unconsciously hold your breath. For example, when I am on top of a ladder trying to hammer in a nail that is slightly out of reach and I dislodge the nail, bang my thumb, or bend the nail, I stop and say to myself, "Baker, stop holding your breath and take a deep one with your diaphragm." Then the nail goes right in. The same is true for threading a needle, looking for lost keys, worrying about finding a restroom when you're downtown with a filling bladder, waiting in line at the bank, or driving on the freeway.

8. Engage in some form of rhythmic exercise at the same time every day, preferably in the afternoon when muscle strength is at its peak and most people perform best. If you can walk, walk. If you can swim, do that, especially if you can find nonchlorinated water to swim in and are strong enough to swim with a good steady rhythm. If you prefer, ride a bike. But whatever you do, remember to breathe in a relaxed way, using your diaphragm, so that the effort of your exercise reinforces rhythmic harmony in your body instead of allowing unnatural chest breathing to interfere with it.

9. Working out to music takes exercise one step farther by permitting you to synchronize your activity with the beat of the music. Of course, the ultimate refinement of exercising to music is dance. If you are ill and unable to move about, then simply listen to music, but really listen so that the music penetrates your being rather than simply acting as a background to whatever you are doing. Some types of music are more healing than others. I asked Millie Grenough, a music therapist and author of *Sing It! Learn English Through Song*, what would be the best choice of music for a person with inflammatory illness.[3] She said, "It can

be anything from Mozart and Vivaldi to favorite Broadway tunes, from long-remembered lullabies or Tibetan chants to your favorite song when you were sixteen. The main thing is that it be music the person loves."

10. Meditate daily to reinforce and integrate your body's rhythms. And if you're ill, use meditation as the platform from which you launch the powerful tool of visualization.

When you dance, you put your whole body's movement into the embrace of something bigger than yourself—the music. When you are fully the captive of the music you are free to receive its blessing. And every step of the dance is a choice you make to stay with the music.

I hope this book has brought you the message that whether you know it or not, you're dancing. You are a participant in a musical enterprise called life, in which the fundamental beat is the day-and-night cycle of the planet we all share. Everything you do has the potential to put you more or less in harmony with this rhythm. In the future, science may bring more complex and precise ways of integrating your body rhythms and living in balance and harmony with our planet. But the Circadian Prescription gives you a piece of the future now.

24:00
25:00
01:00
02:00
03:00
04:00
05:00
06:00
07:00
08:00
09:00
10:00
11:00
12:00
13:00
14:00
15:00
16:00
17:00
18:00
19:00
20:00
21:00
22:00
·23:00
24:00
25:00
0i:00

APPENDIX

A

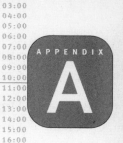

Traveling

TAKING THE SHAKE ON THE ROAD

If you travel frequently, here's an addition to your survival kit for living out of your suitcase. Before you leave, mix together 1 heaping tablespoon of soy protein powder and 1 heaping tablespoon of flaxseed powder for every day you'll be away. Store the mixture in a Ziploc bag or apportion it into used film containers. Pack this mixture along with a plastic teaspoon in your luggage. Although ground flaxseed goes rancid more quickly than whole seeds, this mixture should keep for a week at room temperature.

During your trip, if you're on the run at breakfast time, get a glass of juice, stir in 2 tablespoons (6 teaspoons) of the mix, and chug a lug. Another option is to stir it into a cup of flavored yogurt, which you can obtain at most hotels.

Use the same strategy at home if you're used to skipping breakfast during the weekday morning rush hour. Your morning morale and productivity will be enhanced.

PREVENTING JET-LAG

Following these simple steps (adapted from Dr. Charles Ehret's Argonne Anti-Jet-Lag-Diet) will help you quickly adjust your body's clock when you travel across time zones.

1. Determine breakfast time at your destination and start the diet four days earlier.

2. Day 1. Eat a high protein breakfast and lunch and a high carbohydrate dinner (FEAST). Drink coffee only between 3:00 and 5:00 p.m.

3. Day 2. Eat only light meals—salads, light soups, fruits and juices, unbuttered toast. Keep calories and carbohydrates to a minimum (FAST). Again, drink coffee only between 3:00 and 5:00 p.m.

4. Day 3. Repeat what you did on day 1 (FEAST).

5. Day 4 (day of departure). FAST. On this day, if you drink caffeine, have it in the morning if you are traveling west or between 6:00 and 11:00 p.m. if you are traveling east. When you break the fast, do it with a high protein breakfast if you have a morning arrival or a high carbohydrate dinner if you have an arrival late in the day.

6. Don't drink any alcohol on the plane. If the flight is long enough, sleep, but sleep no later than breakfast time at your destination.

7. Stay awake and active during your first day. Eat your meals according to local mealtimes.

For an individually tailored detailed program to counteract jet lag, see the Web site http://www.stopjetlag.com, which was created in consultation with Dr. Ehret.

```
24:00
25:00
01:00
02:00
03:00
04:00
05:00
06:00
07:00
08:00
09:00
10:00
11:00
12:00
13:00
14:00
15:00
16:00
17:00
18:00
19:00
20:00
21:00
22:00
23:00
24:00
25:00
01:00
```

Shift Work

B

HOW TO HANDLE ROTATING, NIGHT, OR EVENING SHIFTS

Human chemistry is geared to sleep, restoration, and repair at night and the full exploitation of consciousness during the day. Doing things the other way around is not natural, but millions of us do so at some cost to our health and safety. Some individuals are more adaptable than others, who could never function effectively if their work required them to oppose the normal day-night schedule by working at night. Those who have the most challenge to their physiology and health are those who don't work regular day or night jobs but instead have to adapt to periodic changes in the rotation.

Employers in all sectors of the military and civilian economy have used circadian research to learn how they can help workers achieve improved health and reduce the risk of the enormous losses that arise from accidents due to human error. As Dr. Martin Moore-Ede points out in his book *The Twenty Four Hour Society*,[1] the Three Mile Island and Chernobyl nuclear disasters, the Exxon Valdez accident, Bhopal, numerous plane crashes, and countless other catastrophes have all happened at times of day (night, actually) when human functioning is low. Shift work's negative effect on the way we function played a significant role in causing many of those calamities.

Incorporating scientific research and principles into planning shift work rotations is beneficial to health, morale, productivity, and the bottom line. Unfortunately, many employers stick with traditional methods of shift work planning.

Here are some guidelines that may help you negotiate healthier rotations with your employer or at least to adapt when your shift rotations are not under your control.

1. Slow rotation, allowing your body to adapt to each shift as you come to it, is preferable to fast rotation. An example of fast rotation is working day shift on Monday, night shift on Tuesday, evening shift on Wednesday, and night shift on Thursday. In other words, you're working different shifts in the same week, expecting your body to stay on "regular time" while you work at the "wrong time of day."

2. Delayed rotation, in which you move in the direction of morning shift to afternoon shift to night shift (remember: it's MAN) is much better than advanced rotation, in which you move from morning shift to night shift to afternoon shift.

3. If you must rotate, you should stay at least a week or more on each shift.

4. When you are on a shift, you should live the shift. Move your whole schedule so that it conforms to the practices outlined in the following table. It will take a few days to adjust, but it is better to do that than to spend the whole rotation with your body in rhythmic turmoil.

5. Be sure you have two days off between shift changes. Use the table to guide you in preparing for the new shift.

If the shift change is a phase delay (going from morning shift to afternoon, afternoon to night, or night to morning), you can do even better by following some simple rules for preparing. Here are the rules, which depend on two days off between shift changes.

- The times in the Early phase column are the beginning of the work shift.

RULES FOR LIVING THE SHIFT

SHIFT	EARLY PHASE	MIDDLE PHASE	REST PHASE	PRESLEEP PHASE
	✿	○	★	●
Morning Shift	7:00 a.m.	12 noon	3:30 p.m.	6:00 p.m.
Afternoon Shift	3:00 p.m.	8:00 p.m.	11:30 p.m.	2:00 a.m.
Night Shift	11:00 p.m.	4:00 a.m.	7:30 a.m.	10:00 a.m.
Meals	"Breakfast"	"Lunch"	"Teatime"	"Supper"
Activities	• Lights on • Exercise • Big, high protein breakfast • No caffeine	• No naps • Big, high protein lunch • No caffeine	• Coffee, tea, or cocoa • Sweets	• High carbohydrate, low protein supper • No caffeine • Low-key exercise

Source: Information in these three tables adapted from Ehret, C. F. New approaches to chronohygiene for the shift worker in the nuclear power industry. In Advances in the Biosciences, vol. 30, *Night and Shift Work, Biological and Social Aspects.* ed. A. Reinberg et al. Oxford: Pergamon Press 1981, pp. 263-269.

- The Activities in the Early phase column are what you should do when getting up at the appropriate time before work to have "breakfast," and so on.

- The times shown in the Mid phase column should be considered "noon" on each shift while you are at work. For example, on the night shift you would have a big, high protein "lunch" at 4:00 a.m.

- The Rest phase refers to the time after you get out of work.

- The Presleep phase refers to the time and the meal that precedes sleep. If you are on the afternoon shift, for example, this phase would start around 4:00 or 5:00 a.m. and last for eight hours, ending between noon and 1:00 p.m. in time for "breakfast" and getting to work.

- This scheme is the same if you stay on the same shift for more than a week or if you're on a permanent shift.

PREPARING FOR SHIFT CHANGE, PHASE DELAY

TIME	ACTIVITY
Day before last day of old shift	Regular routine
Last day of old shift	Eat heavily
First day off (at the phase times of the shift you are coming from)	Early phase: Eat sparingly and avoid carbohydrates except for a little fruit; drink several cups of strong black coffee
	Middle phase: Continue to eat sparingly
	Presleep phase: Eat sparingly, avoiding carbohydrates except for light salad and fruit; take no coffee or tea except decaf
Second day off (at the phase times of the shift you are heading for)	Early phase: Lights on, big, high protein breakfast; no coffee, tea, or chocolate
	Middle phase: Big, high protein lunch
	Presleep phase: High carbohydrate, low protein supper. Early to bed, new shift time
First day of new shift	Follow the regular routine for the new shift

A phase advance (going from morning to night, night to afternoon, or afternoon to evening) is the less preferred shift rotation but it is still practiced in many industries that took their lead from the watch rotation of the navy. It is backwards according to scientific evidence but deeply rooted in tradition. The preparation is trickier because this is a much more difficult change for your body to handle. The main difficulty has to do with the caffeine intake—several cups of black coffee—recommended in the Presleep phase of your first day off, which may give you a bad night's sleep before your second day off. The tradeoff is that your body's clock will be reset more quickly in order to face the beginning of your new shift.

PREPARING FOR SHIFT CHANGE, PHASE ADVANCE

TIME	ACTIVITY
Day before last day of old shift	Regular routine
Last day of old shift	Eat heavily
First day off (at the phase times of the shift you are coming from)	Early phase: Eat sparingly and avoid carbohydrates except for a little fruit; take no coffee or tea
	Middle phase: continue to eat sparingly
	Presleep phase: eat sparingly, drink several cups of black coffee
Second day off (at the phase times of the shift you are heading for)	Early phase: Lights on, big, high protein breakfast; no coffee, tea, or chocolate
	Middle phase: Big, high protein lunch
	Presleep phase: High carbohydrate, low protein supper. Early to bed, new shift time
First day of new shift	Follow the regular routine for the new shift

23:00
24:00
25:00
01:00
02:00
03:00
04:00
05:00
06:00
07:00
08:00
09:00
10:00
11:00
12:00
13:00
14:00
15:00
16:00
17:00
18:00
19:00
20:00
21:00
22:00
23:00
24:00
25:00
01:00

Glossary

ACROPHASE The time in the circadian cycle when a measured activity reaches its highest (*acro*) peak.

ADRENERGIC Having to do with a branch of chemistry in which the "upper" kinds of neurotransmitters in the adrenaline family are formed. This branch is particularly active during the day.

ALPHA-LINOLENIC ACID The mother of the omega-3 family of fatty acids. It is an essential nutrient, in that humans cannot synthesize it and must obtain it from the diet.

AMINO ACIDS Small molecules made of carbon, hydrogen, nitrogen, and in some instances sulfur. There are twenty-two naturally occurring amino acids that form proteins when hooked end-to-end like a long paper clip chain. Individually, some amino acids are the raw materials for making message-carrying molecules such as peptides, neurotransmitter, and hormones.

AMPLITUDE The height of the wave peaks. Some daily rhythmic changes in humans are very high and sharp, such as the nighttime spike of blood melatonin levels, and some have a low amplitude, such as the gentle rise and fall of white blood count.

CAPP Circadian acrophase for peak performance. For example, the capacity to metabolize ingested alcohol peaks at 9:00 p.m.

CHOLESTEROL A complex molecule used by animals to make steroid hormones (e.g., estrogen, progesterone, testosterone, and cortisol) and as a component of cell membranes.

CHRONOBIOTIC Any drug that is a timegiver.

CIRCADIAN "About a day." In humans the circadian rhythm is a little more than twenty-four hours, and without any signals (light, food, activity) from outside to reset it to the earth's twenty-four-hour day and night cycle, it would run with amazing precision within minutes of its set tempo.

CYTOPLASM The watery material inside a cell that surrounds the nucleus. Mitochondria and other important cellular machinery are in the cytoplasm.

DAIDZEIN An isoflavone found in foods such as soy.

DIGLYCERIDE Two fatty acids joined by another molecule. This is the structure of the fat in the membranes in and around body cells.

DYSCHRONOGEN A drug or other influence that has a negative effect on circadian rhythms.

ENZYMES Large proteins whose embrace brings together or separates other molecules to facilitate chemical reactions.

FATTY ACID The smallest unit of fat.

GENISTEIN An isoflavone found in foods such as soy.

GLUTEN A protein in wheat, barley, and rye. Its imperfect digestion can release peptides that resemble peptides we make for ourselves and that thus become mischievous mimics of our chemistry.

HYDROGENATION A method for treating unsaturated oils so that they become artificially saturated (with hydrogen) and therefore stiffer, less susceptible to becoming rancid, and more toxic.

INFRADIAN "More than a day"—for example, rhythms that cycle in intervals of weeks, such as the menstrual cycle of four weeks.

ISOFLAVONES Molecules found in some foods, especially soy, that have a potential to influence human chemistry.

LIGNANS Plant pigments found in many foods, such as whole rye and flax seeds, that release chemicals that influence human chemistry.

LIPID All fatty molecules that are insoluble in water.

MELATONIN A derivative of serotonin that acts as an antioxidant and message-carrying molecule and whose activities are bound to the dark/sleep cycle of humans. The peak of melatonin levels in the blood at about 3:00 a.m. is one of the sharpest and narrowest of all the body's circadian cycles.

MITOCHONDRIA Cigar-shaped compartments inside cells where most of the energy metabolism takes place. In the evolutionary past, cells with nuclei took bacteria on board to act as their energy metabolism subcontractors. Such bacteria are the origins of the mitochondria we have today. Consequently germs, such as yeasts, which can make poisons to kill bacteria, can also harm our mitochondria because mitochondria still resemble bacteria in some ways.

NEUROTRANSMITTER A chemical that transmits an electrical message from a nerve to another nerve, muscle, or other tissue to which it connects. Neurotransmitters are a subset of informational substance molecules. The use of the more modern term "informational substances" acknowledges that there is not as much specificity as was previously believed to the domains of neurotransmitters (nervous system), hormones (endocrine system) and prostaglandins (cell-to-cell communication).

NUCLEUS The package inside cells where the deoxyribonucleic acid (DNA) is stored. The DNA, in the form of chromosomes, is our ancestral memory.

OMEGA-3 A family of essential fatty acids found in vegetable oils. An omega-3 fatty acid is a chain of eighteen carbon atoms in which the first double bond is three in from the omega (unchanging) end of the molecule. Flaxseed oil contains large amounts of alpha-linolenic acid, which is the first step in the omega-3 assembly line.

OMEGA-6 A family of essential fatty acids found in vegetable oils. An omega-6 fatty acid is a chain of eighteen carbon atoms in which the first double bond is six in from the omega (unchanging) end of the molecule.

OMENTUM An apron of fat that hangs over the intestine inside the abdominal wall and becomes the main place where fat accumulates in individuals with apple obesity.

PERIOD The length of time between peaks of a wave that rises and falls with time.

PHASE SHIFT A resetting of the acrophase to an earlier (phase advance) or later (phase delay) time of day. If you travel from the East Coast to the West Coast of the United States, your body has to do a phase delay after you arrive in order to synchronize your chemistry and performance with West Coast time. Conversely, travel eastward from the United States to Europe requires a phase advance. In general, phase advance is much more difficult for your body to handle than phase delay.

SEROTONIN A neurotransmitter that is abundant in the digestive tract and in the brain. Its levels in the blood typically rise at night and are associated with sleep. Its modulation is a target of a variety of mood-controlling drugs such as the selective serotonin reuptake inhibitor (SSRI) drugs, for example, Prozac, Paxil, Wellbutrin, and Serzone.

TRIGLYCERIDE Three fatty acids held together by another small molecule; what constitutes body fat.

TRYPTOPHAN An amino acid from which serotonin and melatonin are formed.

ULTRADIAN "Less than a day"—for example, rhythms that cycle up and down many times a day—such as breathing sixteen times a minute.

ZEITGEBER From the German (*zeit,* time; *geber,* giver); an influence such as light, activity, food, or drugs that tends to change or reinforce the body's circadian rhythm.

23:00
24:00
25:00
01:00
02:00
03:00
04:00
05:00
06:00
07:00
08:00
09:00
10:00
11:00
12:00
13:00
14:00
15:00
16:00
17:00
18:00
19:00
20:00
21:00
22:00
23:00
24:00
25:00
01:00

Recommended Reading

Baker, Sidney M. *Detoxification and Healing.* New Canaan, CT: Keats, 1997.

Block, Mary Ann. *No More Ritalin: Treating ADHD without Drugs.* New York: Kensington Books, 1996.

Bonny, Helen L. and Louis M. Savory. *Music and Your Mind: Listening with a New Consciousness.* 2nd edition, Talman, 1998.

Campbell, Don. *Healing Powers of Tone and Chant: A Two-Cassette Audio Workshop.* Quest Books, 1994. 306 W. Geneva Rd., P.O. Box 270, Wheaton, IL 60189-0270; 708-665-0130.

Campbell, Don. *The Roar of Silence: Healing Powers of Breath, Tone and Music.* Quest Books, 1989. 306 W. Geneva Rd., P.O. Box 270, Wheaton, IL 60189-0270; 708-665-0130.

Crook, William. *The Yeast Connection.* Jackson, TN: Professional Books, 1986.

Ehret, Charles F., and L. W. Scanlan. *Overcoming Jet Lag.* New York: Berkley Books, 1983.

Galland, Leo. *Power Healing.* New York: Random House. 1998.

Grenough, Millie. *Sing It! Learn English through Song* (texts and cassettes). McGraw Hill-Publication, 1995.

Lingerman, Hal A. *The Healing Energies of Music.* Wheaton, IL: Quest Books, 1983.

Mathieu, W. A. *The Listening Book: Discovering Your Own Music.* Boston: Shambhala Publications, 1991.

McCully, Kilmer and Stacey. *The Heart Revolution: The B Vitamin Breakthrough That Lowers Homocysteine, Cuts Your Risk of Heart Disease, and Protects Your Health.* New York: HarperCollins, 1999.

Moore-Ede, Martin. *The Twenty Four Hour Society.* Reading, MA: Addison-Wesley, 1993.

Pierpaoli, Walter, William Regelson, and Carol Colman. *The Melatonin Miracle.* New York: Pocket Books, 1996.

Regelson, William, and Carol Colman. *The Superhormone Promise: Nature's Antidote to Aging.* New York: Pocket Books, 1997.

Ristad, Eloise. *A Soprano on Her Head: Right-Side-Up Reflections on Life and Other Performances.* Moab, UT: Real People Press, 1982.

Rudin, Donald O. *Omega 3 Oils: To Improve Mental Health, Fight Degenerative Diseases and Extend Your Life.* Garden City, NY: Avery, 1996.

Shaw, William. *Biological Treatments for Autism and PDD.* Vancouver, BC: Sunflower, 1998.

Siegel, Bernie S. *Love, Medicine and Miracles: Lessons Learned about Self-Healing from a Surgeon's Experience with Exceptional Patients.* New York: Harperperennial, 1990.

Siguel, Edward. *Essential Fatty Acids in Health and Disease: Using the Essential Fats w3 and w6 to Improve Your Health, Lower Your Cholesterol and Prevent Cardiovascular Disease.* Brookline, MA: Nutrek, 1995.

Simopoulos, Artemis, and J. Robinson. *The Omega Diet: The Lifesaving Nutritional Program Based on the Diet of the Island of Crete.* New York: HarperCollins, 1999.

Taylor, Dale. *Biomedical Foundations of Music As Therapy.* St. Louis, MO: MMB Music, 1997.

Truss, C. Orian. *The Missing Diagnosis.* PO Box 26508, Birmingham, AL, 1982.

Udo, Erasmus. *Fats That Heal, Fats That Kill: The Complete Guide to Fats, Oils, Cholesterol and Human Health.* Alive Books, 1999.

Walker, Sydney. *The Hyperactivity Hoax.* New York: St. Martin's Press, 1998.

24:00
25:00
01:00
02:00
03:00
04:00
05:00
06:00
07:00
08:00
09:00
10:00
11:00
12:00
13:00
14:00
15:00
16:00
17:00
18:00
19:00
20:00
21:00
22:00
23:00
24:00
25:00
01:00

Notes

INTRODUCTION

1. Ehret, C. F., K. Groh, J. C. Meinert. Circadian dyschronism and chronotypic ecophilia as factors in aging and longevity. In *Aging and Biological Rhythms,* eds. H. V. Samis and S Capobianco. Plenum, 1978 pp. 185–213.

CHAPTER 1. LIFE IS RHYTHM

1. Ehret, C. F. New approaches to chronohygiene for the shift worker in the nuclear power industry. In *Advances in the Biosciences,* vol. 30, *Night and Shift Work, Biological and Social Aspects,* ed. A. Reinberg et al. Oxford: Pergamon Press 1981, pp. 263–269.
2. Halberg F. Physiologic 24-hour periodicity: General and procedural considerations with reference to the adrenal cycle. Z. Vitamin, Hormon-u. Fermentforsch. 10:225–296 (1959).
3. Czeisler, C. A., J. F. Duffy, T. L. Shanahan, E. N. Brown, J. F. Mitchell, D. W. Rimmer, J. M. Ronda, E. J. Silva, J. A. Allan, J. S. Emens, D. Derk-Jan, R. E. Kronauer. Stability, precision, and near-24-hour period of the human circadian pacemaker. *Science* 284:2177–2181.
4. Akerstedt, T. Adjustment of physiologic circadian rhythms and the sleep-wake cycle to shift work. In *Hours of Work: Temporal Factors in Work Scheduling,* ed S. Folkhard and T. H. Monk. New York: Wiley, 1995, pp. 185–198.
5. Monk, T. H. Traffic accident increases as a possible endicant of desynchronosis. *Chronobiologica* 7:527 (1980).
6. Ehret, C. F.. On circadian cybernetics, and the innate and genetic nature of circadian rhythms. In *Chronobiology: Principles and Application to Shifts in Schedules,* ed. L. E. Scheving and F. Halberg, Alphen aan den Rijn, Netherlands: Sijthoff and Noordhoff, 1980, pp. 109–125.

CHAPTER 2. THE PARADOX OF INDIVIDUALITY

1. Ehret, C. F., J. C. Meinert, and K. R. Groh. The chronopharmacology of L-DOPA: Implications for orthochronal therapy in the prevention of circadian dyschronism. In *Chronopharmacology and Chronotherapeutic,* ed. C. A. Walker, K. F. Soliman and C. M. Winget. Tallahassee: Florida A & M University Press, 1981, pp. 47–65.

2. Daly, M. E., C. Vale, M. Walker, K. George M. M. Alberti, and J. C. Mathers. Dietary carbohydrates and insulin sensitivity: A review of the evidence and clinical implications. *American Journal of Clinical Nutrition* 66:1072–1085 (1997).

3. Reinberg, A. Chronobiology and nutrition in biological rhythms and medicine, cellular, metabolic, physiopathologic and pharmocologic aspects, eds. A. Reinberg and H. Smolensky. Topics in environmental physiology and medicine series 1983 pp. 265–300. Van Cauter, E., K. S. Ploonsky, and A. J. Scheen. Roles of circadian rhythmicity and sleep in human glucose regulation. *Endocrine Reviews* 18(5):716–738 (1997).

4. Cahill, A. L., S. M. Ferguson, and C. F. Ehret. Chronotypic induction of tyrosineaminotransferase by (α-methyl-p-tyrosine. *Life Sciences* 28(14): 1665–1671 (1981).

5. Fernstrom, J. D. The influence of circadian variation in plasma amino acid Concentrations on Monoamine Synthesis in the Brain. In *Endocrine Rhythms,* ed. D. T. Kriger. New York: Raven Press, 1979.

CHAPTER 3. FOOD IS INFORMATION: PHYTONUTRIENTS AND NATURAL RHYTHMS

1. Bowman, S.A., M. Lino, S.A. Gerrior, P.P. Basiotis, *The Healthy Eating Index: 1994-1996.* Washington, D.C.: U.S. Department of Agriculture, Center for Nutrition Policy and Promotion. CNPP-5. 1998.

2. Adlercreutz, H. Western diet and Western diseases: Some hormonal and biochemical mechanisms and associations. *Scand J Clin Lab Invest* 50: 3–23 (1990).

3. Nagata, C., N. Takatsuka, Y. Kurisu, and H. Shimizu. Decreased serum total cholesterol concentration is associated with high intake of soy products in Japanese men and women. *Journal of Nutrition* 128(2):209–213 (1998). Draper, C. R., M. J. Edel, I. M. Dick, A. G. Randall, G. B. Martin, and R. L. Prince. Phytoestrogens reduce bone loss and bone resorption in oophorectomized rats. *Journal of Nutrition* 127(9):1795–1799 (1997). Messina, K. N., V. Persky, K. D. R. Setchell, and S. Barnes, Soy intake and cancer risk: A review of the in vitro and in vivo data. *Nutrition and Cancer* 21(2): 113–131 (1994). Kapiotis, S., M. Hermann, I. Held, C. Seelos, H. Ehringer, and B. Gmeiner. Genistein, the dietary-derived angiogenisis inhibitor, prevents LDL oxidation and protects endothelial cells from damage by atherogenic LDL. *Arteriosclerosis, Thrombosis and Vascular Biology* 17(11):2868–2874 (1997).

CHAPTER 4. CARBOHYDRATES: LIFE IS SWEET

1. Adam, K., and I. Oswald. Protein synthesis, bodily renewal and the sleep-wake cycle. *Clinical Science* 65:561–567 (1983).

2. See chapter 2, note 3, second citation.

3. National Sleep Foundation. *U.S. Sleep Survey.* 1999. http://www.sleepfoundation.org/PressArchives/lead.html

4. Irwin, M., A. Mascovich, J. C. Gillin, R. Willoughby, J. Pike, and T. L. Smith. Partial sleep deprivation reduces natural killer cell activity in humans. *Psychosomatic Medicine* 56:493–498 (1994).

5. Lusardi, P., A. Zoppi, P. Preti, R. M. Pesce, E. Piazza, and R. Fogari. Effects of insufficient sleep on blood pressure in hypertensive patients: A 24-hour study. *American Journal of Hypertension* 2(1) (January 1999).

6. Nutrient intakes: Mean percentages of calories from protein, fat, carbohydrate and alcohol, by sex and age, 1994–96. Table 4. 1994–96 Continuing Survey of Food Intakes by Individuals and 1994–96 Diet and Health Knowledge Survey. Agricultural Research Service, United States Department of Agriculture. 1997.

CHAPTER 5. THE BASICS OF CONSCIOUSNESS

1. Friedman, A. Urinary peptides in autistic children. Presented Defeat Autism Now! Conference, Cherry Hill, NJ, October 3–4, 1998. Sponsored by Autism Research Institute, San Diego, CA 92116.

2. Ehret, C. F., J. C. Meinert, K. R. Groh, K. W. Dobra and G. A. Antipa. Circadian regulation: Growth kinetics of the infradian cell. In *Growth Kinetics and Biochemical Regulation of Normal and Malignant cells,* ed. B. Drewinko and R. M. Humphrey. Baltimore: Williams and Wilkins, 1997, pp. 49–76.

3. Fernstrom, J. D., R. Wurtman, and B. Hammarstrom-Wiklund. Diurnal variations in plasma concentrations of tryptophan, tyrosine, and other neutral amino acids: Effect of dietary protein. *American Journal of Clinical Nutrition* 32:1912–1922 (1979).

4. Moore-Ede, M. C. Circadian timekeeping in health and disease, *New England Journal of Medicine* 309:469–476 (1983).

CHAPTER 6. THE RHYTHMIC SHAKE AND THE TEN RULES OF THE CIRCADIAN DIET

1. Anderson, K. E., A. H. Conney, and A. Kappas. Nutritional influences on chemical biotransformations in humans. *Nutrition Reviews* 40:616–171 (1982).

2. See chapter 2, note 3, first citation, p. 293.

3. Potter, J. D., and K. Steinmetz. Vegetables, fruit and phytoestrogens as preventive agents (review). *IARC Scientific Publications* 139:61–90 (1996).

4. Bland, J. S. Phytonutrition, phytotherapy, and phytopharmacology. *Alternative Therapies* 2(6):73–76. (1996).

5. Ehret, C. F., K. Groh, and J. C. Meinert. Circadian dyschronism and chronotypic ecophilia as factors in aging and longevity. In *Aging and Biological Rhythms,* ed. HV Samis and S Capobianco. New York: Plenum, 1978, pp. 185-213

6. The ablation of circadian rhythm by excessive alcohol has not been submitted to formal human studies, but it can be inferred from anecdotal reports and studies in plants

and animals done with alcohol and other drugs that have similar effects regarding their tendency to reset the circadian clock depending on the time of administration.

7. Maher, T. J. and R. J. Wurtman. Possible neurologic effects of aspartame, a widely used food additive. *Environmental Health Perspectives,* 75:53–57 (November 1987).

8. See chapter 1, note 3.

CHAPTER 7. MIRACLE FATS

1. Simopoulos, A. P. Omega-3 fatty acids in the prevention-management of cardiovascular disease. *Canadian Journal Physiology and Pharmacology,* 75:234–239, (March 1997). Geusens, P., C. Wouters, J. Nijs, Y. Jiang, and J. Dequeker. Long-term effect of omega-3 fatty acid supplementation in active rheumatoid arthritis: A 12-month, double-blind, controlled study. *Arthritis and Rheumatism,* 37:824–829, (June 1994). Bagga, D., S. Capone, and H. J. Wang. et al. Dietary modulation of omega-3/omega-6 polyunsaturated fatty acid ratios in patients with breast cancer. *Journal of the National Cancer Institute* 89 (15): 1123–1131 (1997). Udo, E. *Fats That Heal, Fats That Kill: The Complete Guide to Fats, Oils, Cholesterol and Human Health.* Vancouver, BC: Alive Books, 1999. Siguel, E. *Essential Fatty Acids in Health and Disease: Using the Essential Fats w3 and w6 to Improve Your Health, Lower Your Cholesterol and Prevent Cardiovascular Disease.* Brookline, MA: Nutrek Press, 1995.

2. Simopoulos, A. and J. Robinson. *The Omega Diet: The Lifesaving Nutritional Program Based on the Diet of the Island of Crete.* New York: HarperCollins, 1999.

3. Rudin, D. O. *Omega 3 Oils: To Improve Mental Health, Fight Degenerative Diseases and Extend Your Life.* Garden City, NY: Avery, 1996.

CHAPTER 8. INTESTINAL FLORA: SMALL CREATURES ALTER BIG RHYTHMS

1. The background for this phenomenon is explained in Dr. William Shaw's excellent book, *Biological Treatments for Autism and PDD* (Sunflower Publications, 1998). Although his focus is autism, this theory will almost certainly expand to include other conditions.

2. Crook, W. G. *The Yeast Connection.* Jackson, TN: Professional Books, 1986. Truss, C.O. *The Missing Diagnosis.* P.O. Box 26508, Birmingham, AL: 1982.

3. Smith, J. G., W. H. Yokoyama, and J. B. German. Butyric acid from the diet: Actions at the level of gene expression, Critical Reviews in Food Science Nutrition, 38(4): 259–297 (1998).

CHAPTER 9. DRUGS AND SUPPLEMENTS

1. Ehret, C. F., and L. W. Scanlan. *Overcoming Jet Lag,* New York: Berkley Books, 1983.

2. Fernstrom, J. D., and R. Wurtman, Brain serotonin content: Increase following ingestion of carbohydrate diet. *Science* 174:1023–1025 (1971).

3. Wurtman, R. J., F. Larin, S. Mostafapour, and J. D. Fernstrom. Brain catechol synthesis: Control by brain tyrosine concentration. *Science* 185:183–184 (1974).

4. Regelson, W. and C. Colman, *The Superhormone Promise: Nature's Antidote to Aging.* New York: Pocket Books, 1997. Pierpaoli, W., W. Regelson, and C. Colman, *The Melatonin Miracle.* New York: Pocket Books, 1996.

5. Ritschel, W. A., and H. Forusz. Chronopharmacology: A review of drugs studied. *Methods and Findings in Experimental and Clinical Pharmacology* 16(1): 57–75 (1994). Nagayama, H. Chronopharmacology of psychotropic drugs: Circadian rhythms in drug effects and its implications to rhythms in the brain. 59:31–54 (1993).

6. Welch, G. N., and J. Loscalzo. Homocysteine and atherothrombosis. *New England Journal of Medicine* 338(15):1042–1050 (1998); accompanying editorial comment. Oakley, G. P. Eat right and take a multivitamin. *New England Journal of Medicine* 338(15):1060–1061 (1998).

7. McCully, K. S. Vascular pathology of homocysteinuria: Implications for the pathogenesis of arteriosclerosis. *Pathology* 56:111–128 (1969).

8. Smithells, R. W., S. Sheppard, and C. J. Schorah. Vitamin deficiencies and neural tube defects. *Archives of Disease in Childhood* (12):944–950 (December 1976).

9. Baker, S. M. Magnesium deficiency in primary care and preventive medicine, *Magnesium and Trace Elements,* 10:251–262 (1991-92).

CHAPTER 10. BREATHING, EXERCISE, AND MEDITATION: ACHIEVING RHYTHMIC INTEGRATION

1. Hildebrandt, G. Rhythmical functional order and man's emancipation from the time factor. In *Basis of an Individual Physiology: A New Image of Man in Medicine,* ed. K. E. Schaefer, G. Hildebrandt, and N. Macbeth. Vol 2. New York: Futura, 1979, p.19.

2. Stough, C., and R. Stough. *Dr. Breath : The Story of Breathing Coordination.* New York: Stough Institute, 1981.

3. Smith, R., C. Guilleminauault, and B. Efron. Circadian Rhythms and Enhanced Athletic Performance in the National Football League. *Sleep* 20(5):362–365 (May 1997).

4. Atkinson, G., and T. Reilly. Circadian Variation in Sports Performance. *Sports Medicine* 21:292–312 (1996).

5. This principle has not been tested in a formal research project that compares athletes who are entrained to the time they will perform. Dr. Ehret tells me of coaches who have reported the importance of such timing in their athletes, but otherwise this particular aspect of rhythmic integration remains anecdotal, intuitive and logical, not yet experimentally proven.

CHAPTER 11. LOSING WEIGHT WITH THE CIRCADIAN DIET

1. Stolberg, S. G. "Overweight was bad enough." *New York Times,* May 2, 1999.

2. Lerman, R. H. Obesity: An escalating problem. I: Addressing the genetic and environmental factors. *Contemporary Internal Medicine* 9(10):14–22 (October 1997).

3. Ibid, p. 19.

4. Physical Activity Calorie Use Chart. American Heart Association Inc., 1998.

5. Lerman, Obesity, p. 16.

CHAPTER 12. WOMEN

1. Xu, X., A. M. Duncan, B. E. Merz, and M. S. Kurzer. Effects of soy isoflavones on estrogen and phytoestrogen metabolism in premenopausal women. *Cancer Epidemiology Biomarkers, and Prevention* 7:1101–1108 (December 1998).

2. Phipps, W. R., M. C. Martini, J. W. Lampe, J. L. Slavin, and M. S. Kurzer. Effect of flax seed ingestion on the menstrual cycle. *Journal of Clinical Endocrinology and Metabolism* 77(6):1215–1219 (1993).

3. See chapter 3, note 2.

4. About Menopause: Menopause Basics. North American Menopause Society: http://www.menopause.org (1999).

5. Ingram, D., K. Sanders, M. Kolybaba, and D. Lopez. Case-control study of phytooestrogens and breast cancer. *Lancet* 350:990–994 (1997). Messina, M., S. Barnes, and K. D. Setchell. Phyto-oestrogens and breast cancer. *Lancet* 350:971–972 (1997). See chapter 3, note 2. Potential role of dietary isoflavones in the prevention of cancer. Barnes. S., G. Peterson, C. Grubbs, and K. Setchell. In *Diet and Cancer: Markers, Prevention and Treatment*, M. M. Jacobs (ed) New York: Plenum 135–147 (1994). Zheng, W., Q. Dai, L. J. Custer, X. O. Shu, W. Q. Wen, F. Jin, and A. A. Franke. Urinary excretion of isoflavonoids and the risk of breast cancer. *Cancer Epidemiology, Biomarkers and Prevention,* 8(1):35–40 (January 1999). Zava, D. T. and G. Duwe. Estrogenic and antiproliferative properties of genistein and other flavonoids in human breast cancer cells in vitro. *Cancer,* 27(1):31–40 (1997).

CHAPTER 13. CHILDREN

1. "Attention disorder in children still eludes treatment method." *New York Times,* November 19, 1998.

2. Diller, L. H. Running on Ritalin, *Doubletake* (fall 1998): 46–55.

3. Ibid., pp. 47–48.

4. Block, M. A. *No More Ritalin: Treating ADHD without Drugs.* New York: Kensington Books, 1996, and from Dr. Block's presentation of the same name at Defeat Autism Now! Conference, Oct. 3, 1998, Cherry Hill, NJ; sponsored by Autism Research Institute, San Diego, CA 92116.

5. Walker, S. *The Hyperactivity Hoax.* New York St. Martin's Press, 1998.

6. Setchell, K. D. R., L. Zimmer-Nechemias, C. Jinnan, and J. E. Heubi. Isoflavone content of infant formulas and the metabolic fate of these phytoestrogens in early life. *American Journal of Clinical Nutrition* 68(6)S (suppl.):1453s–1461s (1998).

7. Ibid., p. 14595.

CHAPTER 14. MEN

1. Planning for Prostate Cancer Research: Expanding the Scientific Framework and Professional Judgment Estimates. Washington, D.C. National Cancer Institute. June 1999

2. See chapter 3, note 2.

3. Fair, W. R., N. E. Fleshner, and W. Heston. Cancer of the prostate: A nutritional disease? *Urology* 50(6):840–848 (December 1997).

4. Prostate cancer screening. *Mayo Clinic Health Letter* 16(11):1–3 (November 1998).

5. Geller, J., L. Sionit, C. Partido, L. Li, X. Tan, T. Youngkin, D. Nachtsheim, and R. M. Hoffman. Genistein inhibits the growth of human-patient BPH and prostate cancer in histoculture. *Prostate* 34(2):75–79 (February 1, 1998).

6. Carroll, K. K. Review of clinical studies on cholesterol-lowering response to soy protein. *Journal of the American Dietary Association* 91:820–7. (July 1991).

7. Tikkanen, M. J., K. Wähälä, S. Ojala, and V. Vihma. Effect of soybean phytoestrogen intake on low density lipoprotein oxidation resistance. *Proceedings of the National Academy of Science* 95:3106–3110 (1998).

8. Bierenbaum, M. L., R. Reichstein, and T. R. Watkins. Reducing atherogenic risk in hyperlipemic humans with flax seed supplementation: a preliminary report. *Journal of the American College of Nutrition* 12(5):501–504 (October 1993).

9. McCully, K., M. McCully, and M. Stacey. *The Heart Revolution : The B Vitamin Breakthrough That Lowers Homocysteine, Cuts Your Risk of Heart Disease, and Protects Your Health.* New York: HarperCollins, 1999.

CHAPTER 15. CHRONIC ILLNESS

1. Dalgleish. T., K. Rosen, M. Marks. Rhythm and blues: The theory and treatment of seasonal affective disorder. Part II. *British Journal of Clinical Psychology* 35(Pt 2): 163–182 (May 1996). Smolensky, M. H. and G. E. D'Alonzo. Biologic rhythms and medicine. 85(1B):34–46 (July 29, 1988). Muller, J. E., P. H. Stone, Z. G. Turi, J. D. Rutherford, C. A. Czeisler, C. Parker, W. K. Poole, E. Passamani, R. Roberts, T. Robertson, et al. Circadian variation in the frequency of onset of acute myocardial infarction. *New England Journal of Medicine* 313(21):1315–1322 (November 2, 1985). Elliott, W. J. Circadian variation in the timing of stroke onset: A meta-analysis. *Stroke* 29(5):992–996 (May 1998). Smolensky, M. H., P. J. Barnes, A. Reinberg, and J. P. McGovern. Chronobiology and asthma. I. Day-night differences in bronchial patency and dyspnea and circadian rhythm dependencies. *Journal of Asthma* 23 (6):321–34 (1986). Gurwitz, D. Flight attendants, breast cancer, and melatonin. [Letter.] *Lancet* 352(9137):1389–1390 (October 24, 1998). Bellamy, N., R. B. Sothern, J. Campbell, and W. W. Buchanan. Circadian rhythm in pain, stiffness, and manual dexterity in rheumatoid arthritis: Relation between discomfort and disability.

50(4):243–248 (April 1991). Reinberg, A., P. Gervais, F. Levi, M. Smolensky, L. Del Cerro, and C. Ugolini. Circadian and circannual rhythms of allergic rhinitis: an epidemiologic study involving chronobiologic methods. *Journal of Allergy and Clinical Immunology* 81(1):51–62 (January 1988).

2. Siegel, B. S. *Love, Medicine and Miracles: Lessons Learned about Self-Healing from a Surgeon's Experience with Exceptional Patients.* New York: HarperPerennial, 1990.

CONCLUSION. THE TEN STEPS OF THE CIRCADIAN PRESCRIPTION

1. Fries, J. F. Aging, natural death, and the compression of morbidity. *New England Journal of Medicine* 303:130–135 (1980).

2. Vita, A. J., R. B. Terry, H. B. Hubert, and J. F. Fries. Aging, health risks, and cumulative disability. *New England Journal of Medicine* 338(15):1035–1041 (April 9, 1998).

3. Grenough, M. *Sing It! Learn English through Song* (texts and cassettes). McGraw-Hill, 1995.

APPENDIX B. SHIFT WORK

1. Moore-Ede, M. *The Twenty Four Hour Society.* Reading, MA: Addison-Wesley, 1993.

23:00
24:00
25:00
01:00
02:00
03:00
04:00
05:00
06:00
07:00
08:00
09:00
10:00
11:00
12:00
13:00
14:00
15:00
16:00
17:00
18:00
19:00
20:00
21:00
22:00
23:00
24:00
25:00
01:00

Index